Fitness Through Cycling

by the editors of *Bicycling*® magazine

Rodale Press, Emmaus, Pennsylvania

Senior Editor, Ray Wolf
Edited by Larry McClung
Cover photograph by Mark Lenny
Cover design by Linda Jacopetti and Karen A. Schell
Book design by Linda Jacopetti

Library of Congress Cataloging in Publication Data
Main entry under title:

Fitness through cycling.

    Cover title: Bicycling magazine's fitness through cycling.
    1. Cycling.   2. Physical fitness.   I. Bicycling!
II. Title: Bicycling magazine's fitness through cycling.
GV1043.7.F57   1985   796.6   85-2197
ISBN 0-87857-548-0   paperback

2   4   6   8   10   9   7   5   3   1   paperback

Contents

Introduction

Bicycling is a lifetime sport. This isn't just because most people begin riding as children. Adults who make cycling a regular part of their lives generally do so for different reasons than kids. Kids ride for fun, to be with their friends, or because they need transportation. Adults may sometimes ride for pleasure or transportation, but most often, they turn to cycling for its fitness benefits.

Maintaining muscle tone, building cardiovascular vigor, reducing nervous tension, and simply "feeling good" are some of the dividends of regular cycling that attract many adults. Valuable as these rewards are, it's possible to pursue them too strenuously. After years of inactivity, an adult dreaming of a quick return to youthfulness may try to force his body back in shape too rapidly. Then, instead of positive results, he experiences aches, pains, injuries, and eventually boredom and burnout. But if progress toward fitness is accepted as a gradual process, each step along the way can be great fun.

Don't rush into a cycling program or any other fitness program without first assessing your present state of health. The type of health review needed depends a lot on your age and the activities you've been pursuing. Here are the recommendations of Dr. Kenneth Cooper, founder of the "aerobics" system of physical conditioning, for inactive people who wish to begin exercising.

Under age 30: Review your medical history with your

1

family physician and have a complete physical examination within the year you start your program.

Ages 30 to 35: The same, but do so within six months, and add a resting electrocardiogram, or EKG.

Ages 35 to 40: All of the above, but within three months, and add a stress test.

Over 40: All of the above, and a stress test is a must. Also, a treadmill EKG is recommended if one or more of the following risk factors is present: family history of heart disease, high blood pressure, other coronary problems, or diabetes; a heavy cigarette habit.

Let's say you have taken the recommended tests, and your physician has given you the green light. Now just how fit should you try to be? How much cycling should you try to do? A good starting program is 30 minutes of riding *every other* day. Your muscles will feel better after 48 hours of rest so resist the temptation of daily workouts at first. If you decide to become a cycle-commuter, begin by alternating bicycle days with your old form of transportation. As your conditioning improves, you can step up to daily riding, and you can gradually make your rides faster and longer if you like.

Once you have a good base of conditioning, you can move in many different directions with cycling. You can train for and participate in time trials and relatively short road races or longer distance touring events like centuries and double centuries. You might even get ambitious and become one of the thousands of Americans who are engaged in multisport training and entering biathlons, mini-triathlons, and triathlons.

Whatever your reasons for taking up cycling, some basic training principles need to be observed. One that is followed by even world-class athletes is to alternate hard workout days with easy days. Pushing your body to the limit every day will only lead to unnecessary injury and will invite psychological burnout. On the other hand, if you never ride hard enough to raise you heart rate to at least 60 percent of its maximum, you will not experience the benefit of cardiovascular conditioning— the so-called "training effect."

Another rule to take note of is that it is generally better to ride in a gear that allows you to spin the pedals at 80 to 90 rpm than to try to push big gears at a slow rate. The latter is hard on the muscles and ligaments and has been proven to be an inefficient way to use energy. Professional riders, in fact, often maintain a cadence of 100 to 110 rpm. So when you are riding, and pedaling becomes difficult, downshift. When ascending hills, get out of the saddle if necessary to maintain a good cadence. You will never achieve fitness through cycling if you ruin your knees early in your training.

Then there is the important matter of diet and nutrition. Some prominent racers and endurance riders are notorious for stuffing themselves with "junk food," while others carefully monitor every morsel and every ounce of fluid that enters their mouths. Nutrition remains a controversial subject, but increasingly there is a general consensus of informed opinion about what constitutes a healthful diet.

Finally, you will notice that once you get seriously involved in a program of regular exercise, activities that at the beginning seemed difficult will become quite easy. As you get fitter, it will take longer to raise your heart to your training rate, and recovery to a slower rate will come much more quickly. You will find yourself able to ride much longer and more vigorously, and you'll feel better than ever. Eventually, you won't be able to imagine yourself not riding your bicycle. That's when cycling will have truly become a *lifetime* sport for you.

The Editors,
Bicycling magazine

Part One
Basic Conditioning

Shaping Up through Diet and Exercise

An estimated 30 percent or more of all adults in the United States are overweight by normal standards, including a surprising number of recreational cyclists. A good many more are at least a few pounds over their ideal strength-to-weight ratio and paying the price every time they ride up a hill. Excess body fat is not an easily tapped source of energy for exercise, and it takes extra energy to move it around.

So let's say you are a few pounds overweight and would like to shape up. You've thought about going on a diet, but you don't know which one to choose. Perhaps you have tried one or more of the currently popular diets and found that taking off a few pounds is not so difficult, but keeping them off is another matter. One reason for this is that most popular weight loss diets are high in meat protein and low in carbohydrates. Unfortunately, even the leanest meats may be 40 percent fat or more. This means that the high protein diet may actually be high protein and high fat.

You may initially lose weight on such a diet for two reasons: first, fat in food delays digestion, so you feel satisfied with less food; second, high protein intake tends to cause loss of body water. Later, however, when your body reabsorbs water, you regain a portion of the weight that was "lost." A similar thing happens with the use of "weight loss belts," vinyl exercise suits, or diuretics. What you lose is principally water weight that returns as soon as you rehydrate.

6

Balance Is the Key

The major flaw with most popular diets is that they focus on a temporary altering of food intake rather than permanent training in good eating habits. If you eat a well-balanced diet, you shouldn't have to change what you eat in order to lose weight, only how much you eat and how much you exercise. A good diet from a wide variety of whole foods, each eaten in moderation, should hold you in good stead all the time.

And what constitutes a good diet? It is one in which fat is limited to no more than 20 percent of total daily calories and approximately 65 percent of daily calories are derived from carbohydrates. But there are two types of carbohydrates: *simple* and *complex*. Intake of the simple carbohydrates found in sugar and fruit should be kept low. It is the complex carbohydrates found in whole grains and vegetables that are particularly valuable. They break down more slowly and thus provide energy over a sustained period rather than a quick burst of energy followed by the letdown that one gets from simple carbohydrates.

Concentration on complex carbohydrates ensures an adequate amount of fiber in the diet as well. High-fiber foods have many virtues. They reduce the amount of fat deposited in the body, help prevent constipation, and help lower blood cholesterol and triglycerides while elevating high-density lipoproteins (HDL), the type of fat that has been found to be protective against heart disease.

Fat provides nine calories for every gram consumed, more than twice as many as either protein or carbohydrates. This in itself is an important reason for keeping the percentage of fat in your diet low. Since animal protein tends to be high in fat, the majority of protein intake should be from vegetable sources such as beans or other legumes and whole grains. This combination will provide all the essential amino acids. If you do eat meat, emphasize white meats such as chicken to reduce fat intake.

If eliminating fat is the primary issue in weight reduction, just how do you gain or lose it? Fatty acids from fat deposits or from a recent meal are carried by the blood to muscle cells. Inside the cells, enzymes are ready to take the fatty acid apart to produce energy in a process called beta oxidation. Unlike

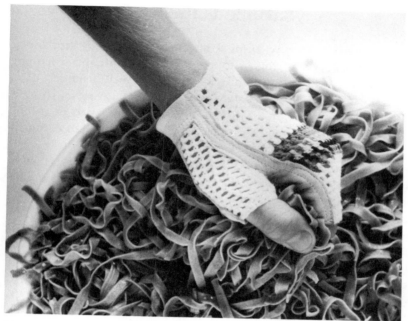

Photograph 1-1. The best diet is one rich in complex carbohydrates, derived from vegetables, whole grains, and pasta.

glucose burning, in which the enzymes require little oxygen in the first stage, all the enzymes used in fat breakdown require substantial amounts of oxygen. Anaerobic exercise (such as an all-out sprint or lifting weights) turns off all fat-burning and forces the muscles to use glucose only. Aerobic exercise, on the other hand, not only allows you to burn fat while exercising but also stimulates production of more fat-burning enzymes.

Here's where a regular program of sustained aerobic exercise comes in: a balanced diet coupled with regular exercise not only increases muscle tone and burns off calories but increases the supply of cellular fat-burning enzymes. Among the best aerobic exercises are running, swimming, and cycling. Of the three, running places the greatest stress on the joints. Swimming has the problem of limited access, since it is difficult for most people to find a body of water with sufficient space for uninterrupted activity available for use year round.

Thus, for many people, cycling is the choice aerobic exercise for getting in shape and staying in shape. Others may prefer a combination of activities: brisk walking, running, swimming, cycling, aerobic dance, and others. The important thing is that you find a way to incorporate sustained periods of physical exercise into your daily schedule.

A Delicate Balance

Weight control really comes down to developing a balance between calorie consumption and calorie use. If you find this balance difficult to achieve, try keeping track of your food intake with the aid of a diet diary. Simply record everything that you eat along with its portion size. You can then check a reference book to find out the nutrient content of the food you ate. One such source is the USDA Agriculture Handbook #456, entitled *Nutritive Value of Foods in Common Units.* This book lists the amounts of calories, water, protein, fats, carbohydrates, and selected other nutrients in a particular portion size for various foods. Such information allows you to make a reasonable estimate of the amount of nutrition you're receiving from your food and can help you discover how you should modify your diet.

"Maintenance calories" are the calories you must consume in order to neither gain nor lose weight. The number, which changes as you change the amount of your daily activity, determines your starting point. In order to "burn" one pound of fat, you must use up about 3,500 calories more than you take in. Once you have established your maintenance level, you can determine how much of a calorie deficit you need to lose weight. You can figure a daily calorie deficit of 500 calories will allow you to lose about one pound per week. If you consider increasing your output by increasing the amount of exercise you get, it is possible to lose weight faster. Of course, if you further restrict your calorie intake, you can lose even faster.

Don't make the mistake of reducing your intake too low for too long, however. You may end up losing protein (lean body mass) instead of fat and also cause serious electrolyte (salt) imbalances that can be harmful or fatal. The generally accepted formula for determining the minimum daily calorie needs of a body at rest is to figure 12 calories per pound, if you are a woman, and 15 calories per pound, if you are a man. Further compensation to lose weight should come from increasing your output rather than limiting your intake.

Increasing Output

To determine your maintenance calorie level you must take into account your daily activity. If your occupation requires heavy manual labor, you are burning more calories than someone who sits at a desk all day. However, you probably are also taking in more calories than an office worker and may still have to exercise after work in order to lose weight. Bicycling may be a good way to accomplish this, in that it consumes about 8.2 calories per minute or about 500 calories per hour (at 12 mph).

In order for bicycling to be aerobic exercise, you must pedal far enough or under enough load to elevate your heart rate to 60 to 80 percent of its maximum for a sustained period of 20 to 30 minutes, three times a week or more. This amount of exercise will allow even a beginner to achieve a "training effect," that is, to start building aerobic fitness. This process will not only increase your calorie consumption and put you in the fat-burning (beta oxidation) mode of energy production; it will also condition your heart, lungs, and muscles.

Actually, increased caloric consumption not only occurs *during* periods of sustained aerobic exercise, it may continue for as long as eight hours afterward. And vigorous exercise helps to decrease appetite, relieve stress, and combat depression. Aerobic exercise also tends to increase the efficiency and rate of fat-burning by stimulating the production of more beta oxidation enzymes.

The Mathematics of Cycling

The average "moderately active," 155-pound man burns about 2,700 calories a day, while a 128-pound woman burns about 2,000. The trick to staying within a desirable weight and body fat range is to meet the body's needs for vitamins, minerals, and other nutrients without exceeding the body's energy requirement. This is difficult for many people, including some cyclists. Having heard that the racer who trains three to five hours a day may need 1,500 to 2,000 extra calories of energy, less active cyclists often assume that they need more calories than they really do.

Figuring your calorie use while riding can help. For example, cyclists burn 8 to 10 calories a minute while riding at 15 mph, or about 500 to 600 calories an hour. The endurance cyclist may consume a great deal of food and drink during an event and still not supply all the energy his body needs, but the weekend recreational rider doesn't train like a racer and can't afford to eat like one.

During the week when there is little time for anything but short rides, the body's energy demands are relatively stable, and it is important to concentrate on eating foods with a moderate to high nutrient density—that is, a diet low in fat and high in complex carbohydrates and with adequate vitamins and minerals.

When you move from inactivity to activity, you need to start out gently. Three workouts per week, with rest days in between, should be enough at first. As you become better conditioned, you may want to increase your workouts to five or six days a week, but always give yourself at least one rest day. And how long should your workouts be? The basic rule of thumb is that to achieve aerobic benefits you must raise your heart rate to the "training" level and maintain it there for an uninterrupted period of at least 20 minutes. Beyond that, the length of the workout depends on the time you have available, your goals, and your level of aerobic conditioning. Remember, when you exercise several days in a row, alternate hard and easy days so that your body experiences a period of stress followed by a period of recovery.

During the week, you may only be able to devote the minimum amount of time to your cycling workouts, but when the weekend rolls around, you may want to spend six hours or more in the saddle, more than on all the other days combined. This is okay, if you work gradually into it. Of course, an increase in activity demands an increase in energy. So, if you like to indulge in cakes and cookies from time to time, this is the ideal opportunity to get away with it when you can use the extra calories.

But remember, the naturally occurring sugars in fruits are an excellent energy source. Fresh fruits have the added advantage of being rich in vitamins and minerals. Figure a medium-

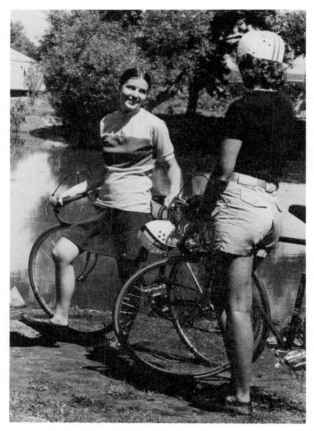

Photograph 1–2. When beginning your cycling fitness program, it is good to find a friend to share your rides, and start out gently, gradually increasing the intensity of your workouts as your level of fitness improves.

size orange, which you can easily toss in a bike bag or stick in your jersey pocket, at 65 calories and a banana at 100 calories. Remember, too, that your body carries stored energy in the form of glycogen so that if you are merely going on a day ride and are slightly over your ideal weight, you don't have to try to eat as many calories as you burn. Experiment to see what sorts of energy foods agree with you when you ride and just how much you need to eat to avoid the light-headedness and lethargy that result from an inadequate blood sugar level.

When Monday morning arrives after an active weekend or when you finish a tour, return to a normal eating regimen so you won't have extra pounds to carry on your next uphill ride. That piece of chocolate cake, which gave you needed energy while you were riding hard, will only flood your system with a surplus of quickly digested carbohydrate subunits when you are following your normal daily routine.

What happens to such surplus fuel? If you are an active racer or long-distance rider, it may be used to replace depleted glycogen stores. But if you are only a moderately active person, your glycogen stores may already be "full up," and the excess simple sugars will be converted to glycerol. This glycerol will combine with free fatty acids to form triglycerides, better known as *fat*, which will then be stored in your tissue.

Finding Your Training Heart Rate

Before beginning any regular exercise program, you need to calculate your maximum heart rate as well as your "training rate," that is, the rate at which your heart must work in order for you to experience the training effect. The first is easy to figure—simply subtract your age from 220. To make the second calculation you also need to know your resting pulse rate. The best time to do this is in the morning just before you get out of bed. Place your fingers on the side of your neck near your windpipe where you can feel your pulse. Count the number of beats in six seconds and multiply that number by ten. This is your resting heart rate, which will probably be between 60 and 90 beats per minute (probably lower if you are well conditioned).

Now use the following formula to calculate your training heart rate. Subtract your resting rate from your maximum rate, multiply the result by 0.6, then add the resting rate to it again. The figure you end up with is the minimum number of beats per minute that your heart should generate for a continuous period of at least 20 minutes if you wish to experience the training effect. Subtract your resting rate from your maximum rate, multiply by 0.8, and add the resting rate again to find the maximum safe rate for your heart to beat during exercise. These two figures provide the target range at which you should aim.

Those of you who are already in good condition may wish to push your cardiovascular system at the upper end of this range; those currently out-of-shape are well advised to aim at the lower end.

Remember, if you have been inactive for more than a few months, you should have a physical examination before beginning any vigorous exercise program.

Some Final Suggestions

You will probably find that increasing your activity is easier than decreasing your calorie intake, so here are some hints and suggestions that may help you achieve a good balance between the two.

1. Don't lower your intake by cutting out meals. Studies have shown that periods of starvation followed by heavy caloric ingestion may increase fat deposition. One giant meal leaves you with more calories available for fat deposit after meeting your energy needs than do several small meals, even though the total number of calories may remain the same over a day's time.

2. If you must snack, choose high-fiber, low-calorie foods such as celery or carrots that will fill you up and not out. It's amazing how much food you can eat and keep to 1,000 to 1,500 calories if you make appropriate food choices. Here's where a book like *Nutritive Value of Foods in Common Units* can prove really helpful.

3. Supplement your diet with a B-complex vitamin, needed for the breakdown of fats.

4. Keep busy, especially with your hands, to cut down on eating simply out of habit or boredom.

5. Walk or cycle whenever you can. Take the stairs instead of the elevator. Every activity over and above your daily routine will contribute to increasing your output.

6. Occasionally, treat yourself to that high-calorie something you've been craving, but do it in moderation and include it in your total calories for the day. There is no reason to feel

guilty about deviating from a strict diet so long as it is an infrequent exception and not the rule.

7. Involve other family members or friends in your exercise program to help your motivation.

8. Be bold and explore new foods, especially vegetables! When it comes to nutrition, variety is the spice of life.

9. Hide your bathroom scale. Check your weight once a week at most, and do it first thing in the morning, after going to the bathroom and before eating or drinking. This will be the least you will weigh that day. If you weigh yourself more often than that, daily variations will only make you frustrated.

Getting Results

Most people who are attempting to get in shape rely too heavily on scales to measure their progress. Be aware that weight measurements can be misleading since lean muscle weighs five times as much as fat. If you are increasing lean muscle mass and decreasing body fat, your weight may stay constant or even increase slightly. Much more important than monitoring weight fluctuations is to use a tape measure and watch the inches gradually disappear or to obtain skin calipers and periodically take skinfold measurements, which reveal percentage of body fat. And don't ignore the more subtle benefits of your conditioning program: the extra spring in your step, your sharper mental alertness at work, your increased energy. Don't be discouraged; positive results are not always noticeable immediately, but eventually you will *feel* them.

Start Your Spring Training Indoors

Every winter, Jeff Paulsen, medical director for the Coors Classic Bicycle Race, wears a special coat. It has no pockets, no collar, and it fits him like a second skin. In fact, it *is* a second skin, a layer of fat insulation built up by a lack of exercise and a hearty love for pasta. "I gained about ten pounds out here (in Colorado) one winter because there was no snow for skiing," he told us. "It took me several weeks of biking in the spring to get back in shape."

Now maybe you want to shed your weighty winter coat early this year. Or perhaps you want to prepare for the bicycle touring season by getting in shape months in advance. You might just be interested in feeling good year-round. Whatever the reason, you don't have to brave snow, ice, and early darkness to get your exercise. There are plenty of indoor alternatives for the winter. Riding rollers is always good for perfecting your spin and technique, and high-tech stationary bikes are becoming increasingly popular. Designed with the advanced cyclist in mind, many come equipped with toe clips, straps, and dropped handlebars. You can also mount your favorite road bike on a wind-load training device for stationary riding.

Whether you prefer recreational cycling, touring, or racing, exercising indoors several times a week will help condition your body for the kind of riding you really enjoy once the road conditions are suitable. But if you skip a few months of working out, you'll have to spend time in the warmer months getting used to being back in the saddle. "Basically, it's a matter of 'use it or lose it,' " says Paulsen. "Skipping a few months of regular exercise is a big setback. It's going to take two months on the road to bounce back."

"You'll definitely see a decrease in your body's capacity to do work (if you abstain from exercise this winter)," says Bill Fink, Ph.D., research associate for Ball State University's Human Performance Laboratory. "Your resting heart rate will start to climb, the capillaries which opened through exercise will close, and the muscle tissue surrounding the lungs will decrease its capacity to transport oxygen."

You can, of course, choose from any number of aerobic sports to keep in shape. You can swim, jog, play racquetball, or attend an aerobic dance class, but many cyclists find that none of these activities can compete with the convenience of cycling in their own homes. Moreover, since exercise is "specific," in that it not only gives you overall toning but builds up particular sets of muscles, the best way to train for riding is to ride.

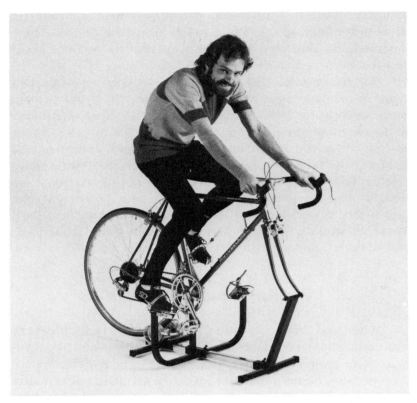

Photograph 1–3. The next best thing to being on the road is to set your bike up indoors on a wind-load training device.

You'll also find it easy to keep track of your fitness progress on an exercise bike. Subtract your age from 220 to get your maximum heart rate, then aim at riding hard enough to bring your pulse up to between 70 and 80 percent of your maximum rate in order to produce a training effect. As you become fitter, you'll probably want to work out with your pulse a bit higher, say 75 to 85 percent of the maximum. You will need to maintain your heart rate within this range for 20 to 30 minutes at a time to realize the training effect. (For a more scientific way of calculating your training heart rate, see the formula explained on page 13 in "Shaping Up through Diet and Exercise.")

The easiest way to take your pulse during a workout is to place a couple of fingers on your neck to one side of your windpipe and count the beats while looking at a nearby clock or watch. If you find this inconvenient, you may wish to invest in a pulse monitor, available through most bike outlets. These devices hook onto your handlebars and are attached to a finger or ear lobe to detect your pulse.

We recommend that even the most experienced cyclists work at maintaining their heart rate in the 70 to 80 percent range in repeated weekly exercise sessions before attempting to do any more strenuous training. Don't begin by cranking the resistance on your exercise bike all the way up and pedaling full force. As Ed Burke, technical director for the United States Cycling Federation, cautions: "Don't start out too fast on a stationary bike. You need to build up your aerobic base by weeks, or possibly months, of steady riding at an accelerated heart rate. These workouts also strengthen your tendons and ligaments so you're better able to try a more strenuous program."

On the Road to Fitness

When you first start stationary cycling, the lack of scenery and companionship may feel odd, but you can—and should—make your exercise bike feel like your road bike. Replace platform pedals with rat traps and toe clips, and put on your favorite brand of saddle. Adjust the seat height so that with your heel on the pedal, there is no more than a small bend at the knee when the pedal is in a full down position. The handlebar height and angle should be adjusted so that when you grasp the hand grips, the upper part of your body is leaning only slightly forward and relaxed, with little body weight supported by the arms.

Begin by developing smooth pedaling form on the bike. Concentrate on making circles with your feet, rather than a jerky up-and-down motion, so you can fully use your leg muscles. Turn the resistance knob to a low setting until you're comfortable with your new exercise partner.

Advanced Training

You know you're ready for something more strenuous when you end each exercise session feeling tired but not exhausted.

You can then start preparing for the cycling season by training your leg muscles to work longer periods of time with less fatigue. You need to focus both on developing *endurance* and *strength and power.*

Endurance is your ability to stay on the bike for long periods of time, the skill you most need for those long summer sessions of touring when speed and strength aren't as essential as just being able to spend time in the saddle. You build your endurance by stressing your body aerobically, elevating your heart rate to the levels we suggested earlier so your body becomes more efficient in using oxygen to metabolize fuel for work.

Strength and power training, on the other hand, involves your ability to perform more intense work for a shorter period of time, drawing on your anaerobic fuel system, which is able to release energy in the absence of oxygen. However, your body can perform anaerobically for short periods of time only. Building your strength consists of developing the capacity to perform a few muscular contractions at a high work load, similar to the brief hard work you experience when you jump away from the pack in a race. Power is strength applied over time; for example, when you're chasing someone or climbing a hill.

Building Your Endurance

Training for endurance is the place to start. This involves long hours of steady riding interspersed with short intervals of fast pedaling against high resistance to stress your aerobic system. Tom Dickson, M.D., medical director for the Lehigh County Velodrome in Trexlertown, Pennsylvania, suggests you begin by maintaining a cadence of 80 to 90 rpm, with a moderate resistance setting, and cycle for an hour. If your bike's handwheel isn't numbered, as it is on ergometers, choose a setting somewhere between the highest and lowest level, preferably closer to the lowest and easiest resistance.

"Ride as much as you can," advises David Smith, M.D., a stationary cyclist who frequently contributes columns to *Bicycling* magazine. "Ride two hours every day for three to four weeks. Work at it intensely; breathe hard. Your pulse rate should be 140 to 150 beats per minute."

Exercise of this type stimulates the narrow, slow-twitch fibers housed in the muscles. These fibers are rich in *mitochondria,* tiny subcellular units that produce energy for the cell through cellular respiration. Mitochondria are rich in fats, proteins, and enzymes and actually increase in number after prolonged steady workouts.

Staying on the bike for long periods of time also helps develop the mental stamina necessary for an extended trip. It may sound extreme, but Lon Haldeman, former cross-country champ, spent many hours in a darkened basement cycling on an exercise bike before beginning his first race across the continent. He not only wanted to build his cycling power and endurance but also prepare himself for the idea of rigorous riding for hours at a stretch. So time in the saddle is always important.

But long hours in the saddle can get boring. Ed Burke suggests that when boredom sets in it is a good time to start doing intervals—specified periods of hard pedaling followed by periods of easy spinning. This will inject variety into your workout and help build your endurance further. "The whole point of doing intervals is to raise your anaerobic threshold, the point when your muscles aren't getting enough oxygen. When that threshold is crossed, the muscle cells start metabolizing fuel in a different way, producing a waste by-product called lactic acid. Once the lactic acid builds up, your legs will cramp and you'll be finished," states Ed.

Naturally, whether you are a time trialist or a tourist, you want to raise your anaerobic threshold. Pedaling at your normal cadence (about 80 to 90 rpm), start by doing three minutes on the bike at a moderate setting but higher than you've been using. Follow with three minutes of slower pedaling. Do ten sets of these.

"Working at this level stresses your body, but not to the point where you build up lactic acid," Burke points out. "Once you've become comfortable with that type of interval program, you'll want to start doing three minutes at a moderate setting, and then a rest period (of leisurely cycling) for only *15 to 30 seconds.* Repeat several times. As you become more fit, you need less of a rest period. Your body is working at only a mod-

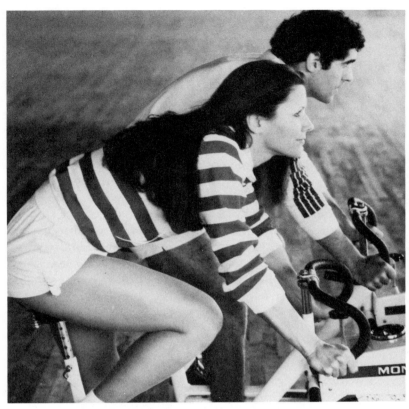

Photograph 1–4. Top-quality stationary bikes can often be found in health clubs and company gyms, where the companionship of other athletes makes long workouts more enjoyable.

erate resistance; you just need about 30 seconds for your muscles to relax before you start again."

Progressing to Power Work

To build your cycling power, Burke suggests doing intervals of a slightly different nature. "Set the bike up at a higher resistance than you did for endurance training, but don't crank it all the way up. Ride hard for 60 to 90 seconds, then pedal slowly for three minutes, to give your body a chance to recirculate its lactic acid and relax your muscles. You need a longer rest period in power workouts than in endurance training because you're pedaling at a much higher work load. Do eight to ten sets of these per workout." Power training should be done only twice a week (and not two days in a row) so you don't overstress your muscles.

Another exercise to increase your cycling power is to set the bike at a fairly high resistance and work hard for two to three minutes. Do four to six repetitions per workout with relief periods (of easier pedaling) of about four minutes in between. You can also build power and strength by setting the bike at a very high resistance, close to maximum, and work for very short periods of time. High-intensity workouts of this nature (and the other power interval workouts) develop fast-twitch muscle fibers that can work at heavy loads but only for a short period of time. Constant repetitions of strenuous work increase the size of these fast-twitch fibers. You can actually see your legs grow bigger with strength training.

Specialized Training

Ed Burke suggests two additional strength-building techniques. The first is *jump training,* which aims at increasing the racing cyclist's ability to break from the pack. Set the resistance on your machine to near maximum, and from a full stop, pedal to your top speed as fast as possible. Then hold the fast cadence for approximately 20 seconds. Repeat 8 to 12 of these in a workout, allowing at least 90 seconds of easy pedaling between repetitions.

The second technique, *sprint training,* also builds your strength. Start pedaling at a comfortable resistance. Then continue pedaling as you adjust the resistance to the maximum. Keep cranking until your cadence drops below 90 or 100. Do this 8 to 12 times per workout, allowing a recovery time of at least 90 seconds after each repetition.

Burke cautions that these strength-building tactics are geared to racers, cyclists who are in top physical condition and usually have a coach or other supervision while training. If you find these exercises too strenuous, modify them. Building your strength and power is relative to your own cycling experience and physical condition. Don't persist in performing an exercise that doesn't feel right. It is always a good idea to start slow and work into a strenuous routine.

One final word about stationary bikes. You may encounter cyclists who insist that road riding is the only way to cycle. But many serious cyclists have found that riding stationary bikes is not only a useful aid to keeping in shape during the off-season, it can serve as a supplement to road riding all year.

Part Two
Prevention and Treatment of Injuries

Don't Let Those Minor Aches Become Major

It was an exquisite day. The Colorado sun warmed the air to a comfortable 65°. Allison Paulsen, wife of the medical director of the Coors Classic, gamely accepted the challenge to ride 60 miles with Davis Phinney, Tony Conforti, and a few other high-caliber cyclists. Her balmy, spring-like outlook was interrupted 30 miles into the ride by a sharp, persistent pain in her left knee. She was to endure that pain, to some degree, for nearly a year. Finally, she resigned herself to a dose of aspirin whenever she trained so she could ride comfortably.

A few months later, trainer Dan Seviers was ritualistically taping Eric Heiden's ankles as he prepared for his first Coors Classic. Seviers was trying to lessen the discomfort of Achilles tendinitis, which was so painful for Heiden that he was ultimately forced to drop out of the last event of the Classic.

As the Coors medical director, Jeff Paulsen sees cyclists all the time with injuries similar to those described. Allison's injury stemmed from a one-time, sudden change in riding habits and a drastic increase in mileage (her fateful ride came after a winter of little cycling activity). On the other hand, the constant, repetitive stressing of Eric's Achilles tendons during his first season of serious competitive cycling resulted in his "overuse" injury. These two failed to remember (cyclists everywhere, take note) that significant increases in training distances and speed are a frequent cause of joint, soft-tissue, and ligament pain.

Preventing Pain

Jeff Paulsen's experience with cycling injuries over the past few years has led him to conclude that the best way to treat pain is to prevent it. He strongly recommends that cyclists enter into their spring training regime gradually. Allison's desire to keep up with a pack of elite riders left her in pain, and scores of cyclists complain every summer of aches and pains that could have been avoided had they been less gung-ho on the bike in early spring. Knee pain, for example, is often a result of doing too much too early in the season.

Mike Nettles, a cycling coach in Boulder, Colorado, has women on his team hold their mileage to 100 miles per week for the first ten weeks of the training season. Not only does this seem to prepare his riders adequately, but it avoids unnecessary injuries as well. Along with limiting mileage, it is a good idea to avoid pushing big gears in the early stages of conditioning. Spin a brisk, steady cadence in a mid-range gear on the flats and stay with low gears on the hills.

You can further reduce the chance of injury by taking other simple precautions. For example, an important part of any cyclist's program is stretching. Stretching makes muscles more flexible and pliable and can prevent strains and aches. The best stretch technique, termed "static stretching," involves assuming the stretch position slowly and holding it for 30 to 60 seconds. In doing so, you will feel the muscle progressively relax, which will enable you to stretch even farther. Do this for a total of 3 to 5 minutes for each muscle/joint combination you are stretching. Don't bounce and never stretch to the point of pain. Pain is nature's way of telling you that something is being hurt. You don't necessarily need to stretch before a ride, especially if you warm up. Actually, the best time for stretching is after a warm-up or a ride.

Muscle-strengthening exercises are also important since weight training is useful not only in preventing but also in *treating* injuries. Many early-season muscle, ligament, and tendon tears, strains, and sprains may be prevented by adhering to a graduated weight-training schedule. Be careful, though, to start out slowly. Too heavy a weight too early in the conditioning program may cause the very injury you were hoping to prevent.

Here, then, are a few words to the wise. After a little warm-

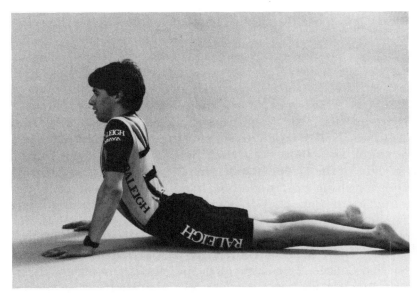

Photograph 2–1. Stretching exercises are very helpful in relieving tight muscles, making them more pliable. Move into each posture slowly, then hold it for at least 30 seconds while relaxing and breathing deeply.

up on a stationary bike or rollers, loosen up with stretching exercises. Stretch again after you've lifted weights. This, among other things, reduces post-exercise pain. Remember, for increasing muscle tone and strength, ten reps with a moderate weight will do you more good than one rep with a heavy weight. Increase by 2½- to 5-pound increments as you are ready. Keep your reps up around three sets of ten each for each muscle/joint group exercised. Be sure to exercise opposing groups equally. Don't, for example, overdevelop your quads at the expense of your hamstrings.

If you are a novice at weights, you really should work out under knowledgeable supervision. A coach can teach you proper lifting technique and help you set up a balanced program that suits your needs. Complement each hour of weight-training with a 30- to 45-minute spin on the road with your bike or on rollers or a stationary wind-load simulator, to keep your legs loose and to reduce post-exercise pain.

Another aid to injury prevention is checking the fit of your bike to eliminate any source of discomfort. Be sure your seat is properly positioned and your stem is the right length for you.

Cleats, if you use them, must be placed correctly on the shoes to allow for your own natural knee rotation—or you are asking for knee pain. And you want to check that the toe clips are the correct size for you.

However, cleat placement is only part of the story for cyclists who suffer from "knock knees," "bow legs," or "flat feet." They may also require an orthotic, a custom-fitted shoe insert. "For cyclists with problems aligning their feet, ankles, and knees properly, an orthotic is a great benefit," says William Farrell, inventor of the Fit Kit, a collection of tools, tables, and instructions for fitting a rider to a bike frame and components. "A flat-footed cyclist like Nelson Vails, for example, generates huge amounts of force on the pedals and requires an orthotic for proper alignment."

Dr. Gibb Hice, Director of Sports Medicine at the Pennsylvania College of Podiatric Medicine, agrees. "An orthotic helps straighten the leg out and influences the relationship of the foot to the pedal," says Dr. Hice. "Cyclists with flat feet, wide hips, and other problems that we've fitted with an orthotic have reported dramatic results."

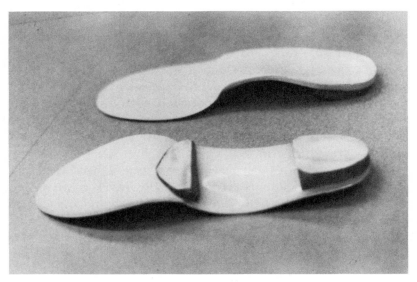

Photograph 2–2. An orthotic, or custom-fitted shoe insert, can greatly benefit any cyclist who has trouble properly aligning feet, ankles, and knees.

Treating Minor Aches

No matter how many precautions you take, there's always a chance you may suffer injury. When skeletal-muscular injuries occur, the program Jeff Paulsen normally prescribes revolves around "relative rest." This means a combination of reducing total miles ridden and riding in lower gears. It takes time to get in shape! This is not only true in the spring, after an inactive winter. It is also true when recovering from an injury. In both cases, you have to give your body time to adjust to the strains you are placing on it.

Depending on the severity of the injury, some physicians may even prescribe *total* rest, meaning a complete vacation from the bike for a few days or weeks. In this situation, switching to another, less stressful sport—such as swimming or walking— can be a temporary means of staying in condition. If you do continue to ride and feel a twinge or two of pain, apply ice to the injury as soon as you can.

The application of ice to injured muscles (cryotherapy) has long been recognized as a valuable treatment for muscle and joint injuries. Ice massage is gradually gaining popularity in sports medicine as it relieves pain and promotes healing by slowing oxygen demands of affected tissues and by slowing the transmission of pain impulses via nerve tissue. Dr. William C. McMaster recommends a 20-minute massage with ice in a peeled-back paper cup to cool deep muscular tissue. Care must be taken to avoid frostbiting or freezing of the skin. If the pain continues with every ride and becomes severe, you'll need to consider a more drastic treatment than ice. Consult your trainer or physician.

A More Radical Approach

The suggestions provided thus far touch on the most common, conservative, noninvasive approaches to injury treatment, which may take weeks to show a healing effect. But what can medical practitioners do for the gung-ho competitor who "has to be back on the bike tomorrow"? In such a case, a cyclist may want an anti-inflammatory drug to reduce pain and promote healing.

The role of these drugs in injury treatment is still hotly debated. Some cyclists, such as Heiden, prefer a conservative approach. He taped his ankles to limit their range of motion, reduced tendon stretch during exercise, and gave the affected joints "relative rest."

For cyclists who opt for drug therapy, under the close supervision of a health care provider, there are several choices, including the nonsteroidal anti-inflammatory drugs (NSAID) and the controversial substances such as dimethyl sulfoxide (DMSO). The use of steroids is prohibited in cycling by the Union Cycliste Internationale, the United States Cycling Federation, and the International Olympic Committee. We can not recommend anyone even consider their use. However, there are other medications you can use.

Oh, What a Relief It Is!

The most widely used NSAID is our old friend, aspirin. In addition to its analgesic and fever-reducing properties, aspirin has an anti-inflammatory effect when taken correctly. "Correctly" means regular, specified doses for an extended period of time. Usually, two or three five-grain (325 mg) tablets every four hours while awake will suffice. But you should discuss the dosage with your health care provider since there can be some undesirable side effects from aspirin use that you both should be watching for.

Advantages of aspirin therapy include low cost and ready availability. Disadvantages include the frequency of doses to achieve therapeutic blood levels. Other NSAIDs are available by prescription only and have their own advantages and disadvantages. On the plus side is the fact that they usually require only three or four doses per day, sometimes even fewer, to achieve relief of pain. However, they are all more expensive than aspirin and require a visit to a doctor's office to obtain the needed prescription.

Intelligent Questions

This is a lot of information to absorb, but knowing it still doesn't make you an authority on cycling injuries, even your own. You may find yourself turning to a physician or, more likely, a trainer or coach for advice. What advice do you need? What advice should you follow? What questions should you ask to assure your understanding of the nature of your injury and its preferred treatment?

Question number one should be "what's wrong?" You want to know what specific structure is involved. Is it a muscle, tendon, ligament, or bone? You will want to know how the injury occurred. Is there anything you can do in the future to prevent its recurrence? Of course, you want to know the treatment for your injury, but you should also satisfy yourself that it's the best for you and your needs and desires. If your coach wants you on NSAIDs, ask why he thinks the other therapies won't work for you. Always ask about the long-term consequences of a particular therapy. And ask yourself whether you wish to shorten your bicycling life by taking a medication that reduces pain and masks further injury, or whether it would be wiser to cool it this season and return stronger next year.

Ask any questions, no matter how silly they may seem. Write them down on paper so that when you see your physician, coach, or other adviser, you remember what you want to know. Don't be shy. You're the one shelling out the bucks. And after all, it's your body and health that are at stake.

Remember! Prevention of injury is always by far the best treatment. Once injured, you can choose among a number of alternatives, from the conservative, safe, and inexpensive, to the extravagant and potentially dangerous. Making the appropriate choice is an individual process, but the advice of an athletic trainer or sports-minded health care provider can be invaluable. If you are serious about your cycling, you really should form an alliance with such a person.

Put Your Legs in Good Hands with Self-Massage

When Felice Gimondi retired at age 37, the Italian magazine *Bicisport* capsuled his racing career with some remarkable statistics. During the 18-year period in which he won the World

Road Championship, the Tour de France, and 143 other major events, Gimondi, rode his bike 551,250 miles, started 2,548 races, and received 2,333 hours of massage. It's safe to say he couldn't have achieved the first two totals without the third. Those 2,333 hours tell us that Gimondi was on the massage table 21 minutes a day every day during his entire amateur and professional career—that he received one minute of massage for every four miles he rode.

The value of massage has long been appreciated in European cycling, where pro teams usually employ at least one masseur/doctor/psychologist called a *soigneur.* In fact, top riders such as Gimondi and current Italian star Francesco Moser often

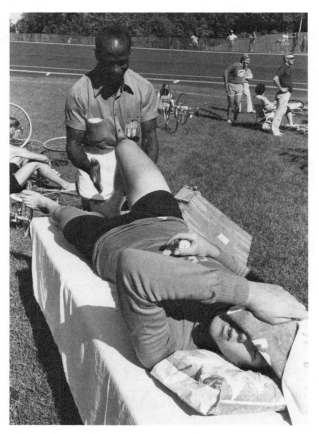

Photograph 2–3. Massage is an integral part of the daily routine followed by elite cyclists.

have a personal soigneur. Moser's is Giorgio Gamberini, who previously worked for Eddy Merckx.

When Moser visited Miami to train for three weeks in January 1982, he was accompanied by his wife, Carla, and also by Gamberini. The fact that Moser was seen with his soigneur almost as much as with his spouse indicates the value he puts on daily massage. Moser accumulated about 2,000 kilometers of low-gear spinning while in the States and spent more than an hour a day in Gamberini's hands.

Also with the Moser party was a fellow named Mario Colosio. A former member of the Italian national amateur team, Colosio, owns a health spa and freelances as masseur for pro teams when they increase their support staff for stage races. In Miami, Colosio and Gamberini gave daily leg rubs to 50 amateur riders at the Moser-led Italia Velo Sport racing clinics. It was an assembly line operation with the cyclists moving through for ten minutes apiece on the table, but it provided strong proof for the benefits of massage.

Firsthand Report

Bicycling magazine senior editor, Ed Pavelka, drove to Miami from the midst of a typically snowy and frigid Vermont winter. His outside riding for the previous six weeks totaled exactly 112 miles. Yet during the seven-day clinic he covered 423 miles during 12 rides. Others from the frozen North chalked up a similar amount. Ed is convinced that daily massage is what enabled them to handle the sudden muscle overload.

When cyclists at the clinic had a particular leg pain, they pointed it out to the masseur. He would nod that yes, he could feel it. He'd set to work on the sore spot, then go over both legs from toes to hips, stroking, rubbing, and shaking the muscles until all tightness left. Walking out of that room, Ed reports, was much easier than walking in, and legs were remarkably free from fatigue during the next ride.

Having hooked everyone on massage, Colosio and Gamberini showed them how to avoid withdrawal when they got back home. The Italian masseurs insisted that self-massage can be very effective on the legs and should be performed as described here after every training ride and race. They stressed that a rider shouldn't feel disadvantaged if he or she doesn't have access to a masseur. Self-massage is far superior to massage from a person who isn't familiar with the needs of a cyclist, they said.

What Is Massage?

What can massage really do for a rider? According to Ed Burke, technical director of the U.S. Cycling Federation, who also participated in the Italia Velo Sport clinics, the main benefits of massage are improved blood circulation and relief of muscle swelling, pain, and tension. It also helps stretch tight muscles and improve their flexibility. Simply put, Burke says, massage is more effective than rest in promoting recovery from fatigue.

Massage will speed relief for those painfully sore leg muscles that often show up after an unusually strenuous, hilly ride or time trial. It is commonly assumed, incorrectly, that this tightness is caused by lactic acid accumulation in the muscles. Burke says it is actually due to microscopic tears in the muscle fibers. Fluid moves into these fibers, swelling occurs, and it hurts. He recommends massage to literally squeeze out the fluid and its metabolic waste products.

The ancient Chinese probably had different physiological theories, but they apparently used massage 2,200 years ago as a means to physical and spiritual health. Theirs is the first written record of massage. Later, when sports were playing a big part in Greek and Roman culture, doctors massaged athletes to improve muscle tone and suppleness prior to competition. After the event, massage was used to rid muscles of fatigue.

The Middle Ages saw massage fall into disuse and even discredit. It didn't become popular again until the early nineteenth century when a Swedish doctor, named Ling, developed a set of rules for massage therapy. After that, a more scientific approach began in Europe that produced refinements in movements and techniques, including sports massage. Today, massage is as much a part of the life of most serious athletes as the tired muscles that make it necessary.

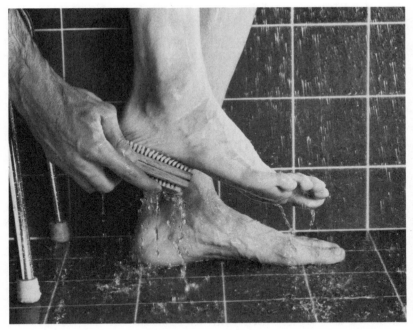

Photograph 2–4. To increase circulation before you begin your self-massage, use a brush to scrub the bottom of your feet while you shower.

Self-Massage

According to Colosio and Gamberini, if you train for racing or simply to improve fitness, you should massage your legs each day. Without massage, they say, you will not gain as much physical improvement from the effort you are making. They advise training after school or work, if possible, so you can relax and do the massage right after each ride.

Use the shower to begin the recovery process. Refresh your body by using cool water in warm weather, warm water when it's chilly outside. "While in the shower, use a brush to scrub the bottom of your feet," Colosio says. "This increases circulation prior to the massage."

After toweling off, put on shorts, shirt, and socks if you like, and stretch out on a bed. Lie there on your back until you feel relaxed, then move near a wall so that your legs can be propped up in a near vertical position. Place a couple of pillows under your head so you can work on your legs without tension in your upper body. This posture should make your legs completely free from tension, and it allows gravity to help pull blood from the muscles.

"During massage you should always use a lubricant on the skin," Colosio says. "There are special creams made for the purpose, or you can use an oil, preferably a natural one like almond oil." (These natural oils should be available in any health food store.) "Of course, to use a lubricant," Colosio continues, "it is necessary for the legs to be shaved. The easy way to do this is with electric clippers (such as a barber uses)."

Once in position, begin working on your thighs. Use steady light strokes with the full hand. Increase the pressure gradually and feel for sore areas that may need a little extra attention in the form of circular rubbing. Then go up to the knee of the same leg and work down from there in similar fashion. Periodically grasp the thigh and shake it for a few seconds, then go back to stroking. When you are finished, lubricate the other thigh and go through the same procedure. Five minutes on each thigh is usually sufficient.

Now slide your feet down the wall until your lower legs are in a horizontal position. This lets you reach the lower leg and keeps it free from tension. Do one leg at a time, beginning at the top of the calf and working down to the end of the Achilles tendon, just above your ankle. Massage the muscles by pressing in with the fingers and pulling toward your heart. Three minutes per leg should do it. Then return to the first position, give each thigh a few more long strokes and lie there with legs up for about 15 minutes.

Finish the procedure by cleaning the lubricant from your legs. The Italians stressed the importance of this, noting that we breathe through the pores of the skin as well as with the nose and mouth. They recommend using a washcloth soaked in rubbing alcohol if the lubricant isn't water-based. Either way, wash your legs with warm water and a neutral soap as the final step.

That's it. The whole routine takes about 30 minutes. It will

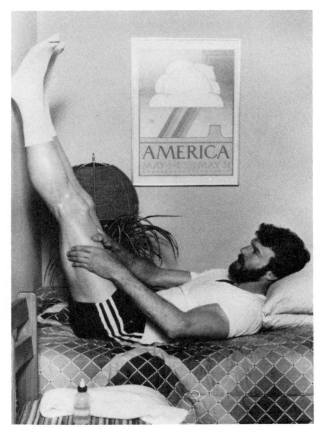

Photograph 2–5. Position 1: Elevate your legs to free them from tension and allow the force of gravity to drain blood from the muscles. Start the massage in the middle of the thigh, working down toward the knee.

effectively empty your leg muscles of waste-laden fluids; it helps remedy specific sore spots; and it gives you a chance to relax. When you ride the next day, you'll notice the difference.

If you must train in the morning and then dash off to daily activities, Colosio suggests the massage will still be beneficial if done in the evening before going to bed. No matter what, he says, "Don't skip it. Massage is very important."

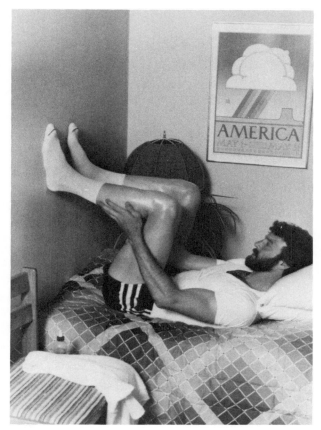

Photograph 2–6. Position 2: Drop your feet down even with your knees so that you can reach your lower legs. Work from the top of your calves down to your Achilles tendons, always stroking toward your heart.

Weight Training as a Way to Prevent Injuries

Bill "the Board" Walters lies facing the floor and tries to raise his upper body with his forearms. He finds it nearly impossible. Although 35 years of cycling have left him in good shape for the track—he recently won a silver medal in the match sprints for his age group (45–49) at the Nationals—his muscles are so stiffened by constantly crouching forward that it's hard to fully arch his back.

"Tied up in knots again?" asks George Hummel, a former world-ranking power lifter who spent three winters coaching racers from the Lehigh County Velodrome (Trexlertown, Pennsylvania) in the fine points of weight training. "I don't think we'll ever be able to straighten you out completely," he says. Hummel recommends some gentle lifts to help Walters stretch and alleviate the pain and then shakes his head in frustration. He is convinced that Walters could have avoided a back injury altogether had he supplemented his regular riding program with lifting weights.

"Ninety-nine out of one hundred cyclists who come to me need to develop muscular strength and mobility in their lower back," he says. "Using weights, they'll prevent back problems ten to fifteen years down the road. But it's hard to convince them to take a break from the bike occasionally." One reason is that it has long been an article of faith that the only way to train for the bike is on it.

Change in Thinking

We now know better. While riding is obviously the most important way to train for cycling, there are also benefits to be gained through weight training. It builds strength and endurance, increases flexibility (when done properly), and prevents injuries. In fact, weight training is considered so beneficial that a regular program during the off-season (November to March) is standard procedure for cyclists at the Olympic Training Center (OTC) in Colorado Springs. Coaches became particularly interested in the training effects of lifting after observing the East German cyclists, who rely heavily on weights to build strength.

An additional incentive to cyclists has been the advent of circuit weight training—a program that not only helps the rider build the strength commonly associated with weight training but maintains or improves aerobic fitness, as well. Briefly described, the "circuit" consists of exercise stations—Hummel's has 16—usually including Universal, Nautilus, or Cam II progressive resistance machines; free weights; and floor space for calisthenics. Participants work in 30-second bouts at each station, moving quickly from one to the next to keep the heart rate elevated and to achieve maximum aerobic benefits. They start by using light weights (no more than 50 percent of a maximum lift) for a given number of "reps" (repetitions), usually 8 to 12 at each station. Going once through all the stations is called a "set."

The riders who work with Hummel swear by the circuit. They claim to feel not only stronger and fitter, but better able to jump on the bike come spring. "When cycling, you're in a fixed position and not really using all your muscles," adds veteran track rider Nancy Kaiser. "Weight training makes me feel more fluid. When I do ride, I feel more a part of the bike." Circuit training offers psychological benefits as well. "Winter always meant spending long, monotonous months on rollers or a stationary bike. Just going to a gym was a big boost," Walters says, claiming he finally took up circuit training after doing calisthenics at home and banging his head on a basement beam. "Weight training was actually a lot less hazardous to my health."

The Aerobic Controversy

The actual aerobic benefits of circuit weight training are still a matter of debate among scientists. In 1976, Lawrence Gettman, Ph.D., formerly the executive director of the Institute for Aerobics Research in Dallas, Texas, was among the first to observe the circuit in a laboratory setting. For five years, he performed studies using over 70 volunteers who were divided into two groups. The first worked through a ten-station circuit in a 30-second work-rest pattern for a maximum of three times. The second group followed the same program but with one difference: participants ran one lap after exercising at each station instead of resting. Not surprisingly, the group that ran laps showed more gains in cardiovascular fitness over the months.

Interestingly, over the years the groups that trained through the circuit without running laps increased their fitness, but no one was sure why. In 1976, volunteers scored less than 10

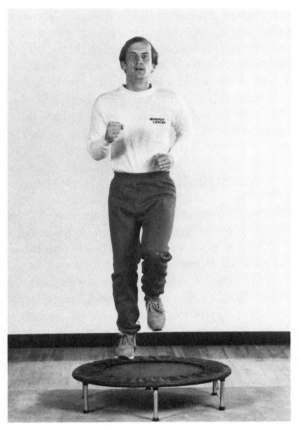

Photograph 2–7. Many circuit programs alternate 30 seconds of running in place, skipping rope, or some other aerobic activity with 30 seconds of weight lifting to maximize cardiovascular conditioning.

percent improvement in aerobic fitness, yet by 1981, that figure had jumped to 17 percent. These levels were determined by a VO_2 max test, which measures the amount of oxygen a person can assimilate in a minute.

Gettman, who previously had considered circuit training to be of little aerobic benefit, admitted he was puzzled at first. "After all, every year there was a new group of volunteers, all of whom had led sedentary lives. Then we discovered that our subjects were growing more fit because we became better at designing the circuit. We put the stations closer together so less time elapsed between exercises, which kept the volunteers' heart rates elevated." So it became clear that to lift weights aerobically, the main priority isn't how fast or how much weight you lift, but how much time you take between stations. The more quickly you move from station to station, the better the aerobic workout.

No Substitute for Cycling

Gettman said, however, that while they proved circuit weight training can be aerobic, it still does not provide the high level of aerobic fitness that can be had through regular running or cycling. It is especially important, then, for a cyclist to find some other sport to pursue in the wintertime, when conditions prohibit outdoor riding. Cross-country skiing, speed skating, or riding a stationary bike indoors coupled with circuit training is much more beneficial than the circuit alone. "We see the circuit primarily as a supplement to regular aerobic exercise," said Gettman. "During a cold or rainy season, you can do the circuit to prevent losing your aerobic capacity."

George Hummel agrees. "The circuit is good for recreational riders because it builds fitness by elevating your heart rate. But at our gym, we meet only twice a week. The other workout sessions are devoted to any aerobic sport the cyclist likes."

The hard fact is that some will improve more than others in their aerobic fitness while training on the circuit. Gary Rollman, 26, a Category II racer, says that circuit weight training gave him a sense of overall conditioning he'd never thought possible to achieve with weights. "Before I started lifting during the winter, I'd start serious training in the spring and get winded quickly. But VO_2 max tests taken over my weeks of circuit weight training showed I had significantly improved. What it comes down to is that I moved fast from station to station and worked hard. That got my heart rate up and helped me get fit. And in the spring, I hardly felt winded at all."

Getting Strong Now

Aerobic conditioning is not the only value of circuit weight training; equally important is the development of muscular strength. "You can have the biggest lungs in the world, but if you have toothpick arms and legs, you're not going to go too far," says Hummel. "For good cycling, you've got to train all the muscle groups."

One area in which cyclists are notoriously weak is the upper body, says Hummel. Canadian coach Norman Sheil agrees. "Recreational riders get very tired on long rides. The back starts to ache; so do your neck muscles and arms. Basically, it's because those muscles are supporting your weight. If you strengthen them, this will enable you to ride that much longer before fatigue sets in," explains Sheil, who worked for years with such cycling greats as sprinter Gordon Singleton.

"Gordon lifted a tremendous amount of weights. I saw that he was able to pedal at high gears more effectively, and he was also able to start faster. Imagine for a moment, Gordon at the starting line. He wants to jump his bike away from almost standstill. Think of the amount of mass he has to move to do that! The stronger he is, the more quickly he can get to full speed." Years of squats and bench presses to strengthen both his upper and lower body paid off for Gordon. He was Canadian sprint champion ten times.

There are some riders, however, who shy away from weight training, claiming they don't want to carry any more muscle than they have to. But circuit weight training does not build extreme bulk since its combination of light weights and moderate number of reps increases the blood flow to the muscles and only allows the muscle fibers to increase in diameter to a small extent. To turn yourself into an Arnold Schwarzenegger, you'd have to lift much heavier weights with fewer repetitions. If anything, circuit training helps you lose excess flab. "My hips were always comfortably padded, even during the hardest part of the training season," says Nancy Kaiser. "But now I'm firmer and leaner. My clothes fit better, too."

But don't think weight training alone will keep you lean. If you eat like a sumo wrestler, you'll soon resemble one. "In

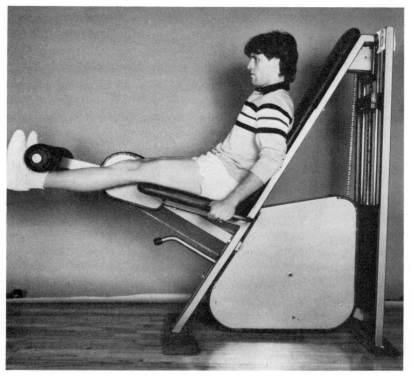

Photograph 2–8. The best way to begin weight training is with progressive resistance machines. They are easy to adjust and less likely
to be a cause of injury than freeweights.

my years of cycling and weight training, I've never put on too
much muscle in the winter," says Dave Tellier, technical man-
ager of the Lehigh County Velodrome. "But I've seen riders start
lifting, stop cycling, and eat like horses. And they wonder why
they got bulky."

Freeweights vs. Nautilus

The question in building strength is how to go about it.
Not all coaches agree as to whether one should include both
freeweights and progressive resistance machines in a circuit
routine. Certainly, working with freeweights has its advantages:

handling the weight properly demands a sense of balance and coordination and in turn gives the kind of overall conditioning that Nautilus and the like—which run on a system of cams and pulleys to exercise specific muscles—can't provide. "When you do a squat with freeweights, you aren't just exercising the chest muscles, but the shoulders, arms, neck, hips and buttocks, too," says Hummel.

But there are dangers, as well as special benefits, with using freeweights. Tom Dickson, M.D., medical director for the Lehigh County Velodrome, recalls a few years ago when the racers first started training, and Hummel hadn't yet signed on as coach. "We thought the cyclists could start on the freeweights doing what's called a 'deadlift'—a maneuver in which you bend over,

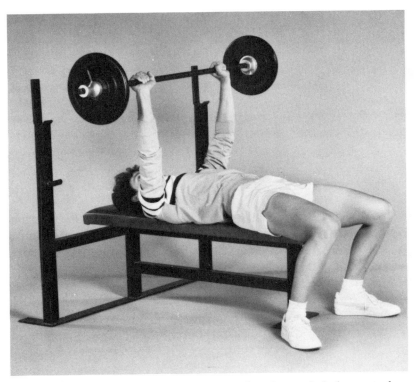

Photograph 2–9. Working with freeweights demands balance and coordination and produces a more complete conditioning than that acquired from only using progressive resistance machines.

keeping your legs straight, and try to lift big weights. And everyone would end up throwing their backs out." Dickson discovered—and every weight-training coach we spoke with agreed—
that the place to begin in weight training is on the progressive
resistance machines. Once comfortable with the equipment and
the lifting techniques, the riders can then integrate freeweights
into their routine. "There's much less chance of hurting yourself
on those machines," says Nancy Kaiser. "The weights can't fall
on you and are easily adjustable to prevent the weight from
causing muscle tears and other signs of strain."

But having the proper coaching is extremely important
with both freeweights and the machines. "If a person isn't sure
what he or she should be using, we'll take a half hour and
establish their strength level," says Hummel. "We'll try different
stacks of weights—20, 30, 40 pounds—and when the individual
starts failing or losing form, then we cut back."

Hummel takes his coaching role quite seriously. He watches
carefully to make sure his athletes lift properly and also attempts
to motivate them to reach down deep when the going gets
tough. "Weight training requires concentration and the desire
to do well," he says. "I can always tell which cyclists are the
gritty ones that will excel on the circuit—they're the ones with
fire in their eyes."

Injury Prevention and Cure

Weight training can help prevent injuries in more ways
than one. Cyclists who train intensively with weights gain a
flexibility and strength that helps them maintain their balance
and control of their bikes in situations where accidents are likely
to occur. When accidents do happen, the upper body strength
gained from weight training can help cyclists absorb the shock
of falling, thus reducing their chances of serious injury.

Then there are injuries that occur not because of accidents
but because of overstressing one set of muscles in relation to
others, the cause of many injuries involving the knees. Resistance machines that target a particular muscle group can be used
to counteract muscle imbalances caused by intensive cycling
and can thus help prevent overuse injuries.

When injuries do occur, whatever the cause, weight training can serve as an important element in a gradual program of muscle rehabilitation. By drastically reducing the normal amount of weight used, you can begin the process of exercising sore and weakened muscles, slowly nursing them back to health. And if you sustain an injury, such as a broken collarbone, which prevents you from exercising some parts of your body, you can still work to maintain strength and, to some degree, aerobic fitness by using resistance machines to exercise the parts of your body that remain uninjured.

Part Three
Getting in Shape for Racing

Training for the Beginning Racer

If you've had a desire to take up racing, but have been afraid of the monstrous miles required to compete, take heart. Nationally ranked riders may put in 500-mile weeks, but you don't have to train or compete on their level.

As a beginning racer, you can learn to be competent without dedicating your whole life to the sport. Category IV races (local races for men who have been racing less than one year) and most races for women are between 15 and 30 miles in length, so there is no need to ride 500 miles a week. It's possible to be competitive while putting in only half that number of training miles. If you want to race, but can't devote five to six hours a day to training, then the program described here is meant for you.

Goals and Base Miles

Establishing realistic goals at the beginning of the season is important. Nothing can be more discouraging than setting a goal too high and not achieving it. If you enter your first race expecting to win, you may be disappointed. It's better to get a few races behind you before setting demanding goals.

If you are a cyclist holding a full-time job, when do you train? For starters, your commute to and from work is time better spent in the saddle than on the seat of your pants in a car. It's a training opportunity you shouldn't pass up, even though it means rising earlier in the morning. If you have to get up at 5:30 and be out on the road by 6:15 every morning, you'll soon find out how badly you want to race.

To get a good training ride, plan a commuting route that is about 20 miles long. Stretch your legs well before you get on your bike and use the initial 15 to 20 minutes of your ride as warm-up, spinning in a low gear at 90 rpm or a little more. After the warm-up, maintain your cadence while you work into higher gears. As your conditioning improves over the weeks, you should work up to 100 rpm or more (after warm-up) in the largest gear you can handle. The primary goal during your initial 1,000 miles of training should be developing spin and laying the foundation for a solid base of aerobic fitness.

Once your spin is developed and you have your 1,000-mile base, you can add hard anaerobic training to your program, but limit really hard workouts to only two or three days per week, alternating hard and easy days. Bear in mind that easy days are as important in your training as hard days because the stress of training, work, and family obligations all take a toll on your body. Easy days allow you recovery time from the rigors of training. Otherwise, your body will revolt and break down from overwork. You can still ride your usual commute on easy days, but you should only spin low gears.

Learn to recognize the symptoms of overtraining since you will probably overtrain at one time or another. Signs to look for are a high resting heart rate, waking frequently at night, and a real dread at the thought of training. Your legs tend to feel heavy while riding, and you just can't spin anymore. You feel perpetually tired instead of strong. Keeping a training log and recording your mileage and progress as well as how you feel will help you spot these symptoms.

Hard Training Puts the Edge On

Your hard training should consist of intervals, time trials, club racing, long steady distance, and hill work. If you can, ride with a group that's serious about training because a group is automatically competitive and will push you much harder than if you ride alone. Don't be scared off because of your lack of experience, give it a try.

Intervals are essential in developing speed and strength. Do them at 75 to 80 percent effort for a given time or distance followed by an equal time of rest—for example, three minutes "on" followed by three minutes rest, then repeat again and again. During the rest period of an interval, continue to ride at 90 rpm but in a smaller gear. This allows the lactic acid in your legs to dissipate more rapidly and gives you recovery time to enable another good effort on your next interval. Do as many as possible until you reach your destination.

On your return trip, try working on sprints. Get out of the saddle for a 100 percent effort for 30 seconds, then settle back for 2 or 3 minutes rest. Do maybe six sprint intervals, followed by a steady spin the rest of the way home. Intervals are very hard mentally as well as physically, so it's a good idea to vary them to keep yourself mentally fresh. By using the same route daily, you can establish landmarks of varying distance as an alternative to riding by the clock. Use a gear that allows you to spin at 90 rpm or better. As your strength develops, you can

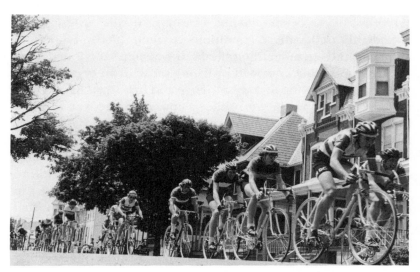

Photograph 3–1. If you live near a racing club, by all means join and race as often as you can. Ask questions and pick up pointers from the more experienced riders.

increase the intensity and duration of each session. Generally, intervals should be done only once or, at most, twice a week; avoid doing them two days in a row.

Although anaerobic strength is essential, the capacity to ride alone at a hard, sustained pace is also vital for racing excellence. The ability to bridge gaps, sustain a solo attack, or get back to the pack after a flat or crash is developed through *time trialing*. Time trials can be of any length, but club events are usually 5 to 10 miles, a distance that riders of all ages and abilities can handle. In sanctioned racing, 25 miles is the standard. The time trial should be ridden at a hard, sustained pace so that you have little energy left when you cross the finish line. You don't want to blow up before you reach the finish, nor should you have enough left for a sprint.

A good way to evaluate your progress is through weekly competition in *club races.* If you're fortunate enough to live near a racing club, by all means join. By keeping your eyes and ears open, you'll learn the finer points of racing. Ask questions, use common sense, and listen to the advice of the experienced riders. Fast riding in a group can often be very shocking to the first-time rider, but the ability to ride at 30 mph in a group, elbow-to-elbow and wheel-to-wheel, without fear and panic is essential for successful racing. Learning to ride skillfully and confidently under these conditions is much safer in club races among friends than learning the hard way in a sanctioned race.

Racing with a club will provide you with an excellent opportunity for getting in *long mileage* and *hill work*. If you race in the evening, put in your miles as usual on the way to work but in a gear you can spin easily. Your legs won't be stressed, and you will be able to race in the evening without difficulty. If you race on a weekend morning, consider riding your bike to the starting line and then home after the race. The ride to the race will serve as a good warm-up, and the ride home can add to your aerobic fitness or serve as a cool-down. A club that engages in racing events twice a week can provide Category IV riders and many women more than ample mileage for aerobic fitness. If you don't have time for this much riding, you can still get by, but if you can find the time, it will provide you with valuable training for sanctioned races.

Although most criteriums are flat, occasionally there are

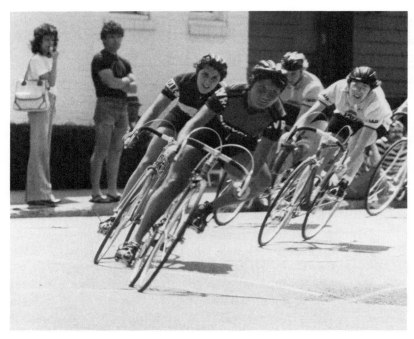

Photograph 3–2. Fast riding in a close group can be very shocking to a novice rider, especially when going around tight corners. It is best to learn this skill among friends and riders whose behavior you can predict.

hilly sections in a race. Therefore you should be prepared for them by including hill work in your training. If your club races on a hilly course, count yourself fortunate. If not, find some hills and train on them for an hour once a week. As with the rest of your training, you should start gradually, climbing in small gears, but eventually build up to as large a gear as you can handle. Remember, in races, you can't rest when you reach the top of a hill. Many times an attack is initiated at this point when everyone is still hurting from a hard climb. If you become a good climber, hills may be the place where you can break away.

Once you have that good aerobic, 1,000-mile base, a quality effort is more beneficial than long slow miles. During the racing season, if given the choice between a hard 15 miles or 30 miles at touring speed, go hard for 15 miles, but be sure to incorporate intervals, time trials, club racing, long steady distance, and hill work in your training week. Don't forget to include some alternate easy days, especially the day before a race when you should limit yourself to no more than 20 fairly slow miles and one interval.

Bike racing is not for the faint-hearted, but using these basic training techniques, hard work, and a modest amount of dedication, you can become a competent racing cyclist. Even if you never win any races, the effort can be satisfying and will help keep your body lean and fit.

Sample Training Week for the Beginning Racer

Sunday: Ride a race or about 40 miles with a group. Work on technique and try to stay with faster riders.

Monday: This is a recovery day from Sunday's race, so keep gears low as you work on skills. Ride an easy 15 to 20 miles in low gears. Work on your spin and smooth pedal stroke as well as cornering technique. Find a short (half-mile) circuit in a suburban housing development or a course in a large parking lot that enables you to go around light posts or pylons. Practice cornering swiftly without losing momentum, and try to ride with others occasionally so you can become comfortable while cornering in a group.

Tuesday: Cycle 25 miles. The first ten should be a warm-up. Pedal easily in progressively larger gears until you are working hard the last mile or so. Then do a series of intervals. Measure them by riding as fast as possible for four telephone poles while still maintaining good form. Then spin easily in a lower gear until your breathing returns almost to normal. Repeat the process, with efforts ranging in length from two telephone poles to six or eight. Start with three repetitions and work up to around ten.

Because quality is more important than quantity, be sure you give 100 percent effort each time, but remember that you won't gain anything if you are fighting the bike and pedaling squares instead of circles. Aim for a smooth application of power during all phases of the pedal motion no matter how tired you get. Cool down during the last 5 miles of the ride by reversing the warm-up procedure. For variety, ride a half-mile hill several times in succession, or mark 100-yard to 1-mile courses on your favorite training routes and time yourself for five or six of them. Compare your times over a season to gauge your improvement.

Wednesday: Spin easily for 15 or 20 miles. This is a recovery day so don't push.

Thursday: Ride 25 miles. Warm up as on Tuesday, and then do a 3- to 10-mile time trial. Use the same course each week and time yourself to see whether you are improving. Beware of over-gearing. Choose a modest ratio that allows you to keep your cadence near 100 rpm. Indiscriminate use of big gears will not remedy poor style or fitness but may cause strained ligaments or tendinitis. Training time trials are tough so try to get several riders together to encourage each other.

Friday: Rest day.

Saturday: Ride 20 miles, spinning easily.

Preparing to Ride Your First Century

Now that you have embarked on a program of fitness through cycling, you are probably looking for ways to bring variety into your workouts. You find riding alone somewhat boring and think it would be fun to occasionally get involved in a group ride, maybe even a race. But, elbow-to-elbow and wheel-to-wheel riding in fast road races is not really your thing. Something a little more laid back would suit you better—perhaps a long distance event, like a century or double century.

Though these events are commonly termed "races," at the outset you should approach them as long training rides. On your first century, you should not be competing with anyone else but simply trying to finish the 100 miles. Remember, whatever time it takes you to finish will be a personal record so don't try to set any speed records your first time out. Avoid the mistakes described by Walter Ezell, editor of *American Wheelman* magazine in an account of his first 100 miler:

"My first century ride was a textbook example of how *not* to do it. Dawn came too early, and running late, I grabbed a couple of slices of leftover pizza and ate them en route to the starting point. (Pizza, I would learn, is hardly the breakfast of champions.)

"As I joined the group in the parking lot, in spite of my newness at this, I felt confident—perhaps too confident. To complicate matters, there stood Andy Anderson, a tall, tan, muscular rider, looking every inch like Hermes, the Greek god of speed. Andy is a bikie's bikie, a fellow that many of the club members would have followed to hell in an effort to keep up. Little did I realize that was what I would do that day.

"I hung on his every word and, flattered by his attention, tried to keep his steaming pace. 'I don't know how much longer I can ride like this,' I finally gasped after about a dozen miles.

'Do you want to go faster?' Anderson asked innocently.

"I let Andy go his own way and I settled into a more moderate pace. About 60 miles into the ride I developed leg cramps, and from then on the century was a real struggle. Toward the end I totally ran out of steam, and two kind but bewildered women in a Lincoln Continental pitied my pleading and hauled me and my bike the final four miles to the campground."

Now that he has ridden many centuries, Ezell says he is convinced that the first one does not have to be a disaster. If you train for the distance, eat well, and ride conservatively, you can actually feel fresh at the end of your ride. Follow the principles outlined in this chapter and see for yourself.

The Importance of Pacing

When you begin training for a century, don't jump into heavy mileage all at once. Start with a comfortable number of miles and gradually increase your distance over a period of weeks (see the suggested schedule at the end of this chapter). This way you will strengthen your cardiovascular system along with your muscles. As your training progresses, pay close attention to the way your body responds. What foods agree with you? What is a comfortable pace for you? How often should you stop to rest? Also think about the equipment you need to make your ride go smoother. Regular riding will provide you with both the self-knowledge and the physical conditioning that will allow you to ride a century without misery.

Long-distance rides force people to be selfish about their pace. If you try to follow someone else's pace for hours at a time, chances are it will either be too fast or too slow. You will either become exhausted before the end of the ride or your rear will want to know why it spent so much extra time on the saddle while your legs dawdled. Find the pace that is right for you and stick with it.

Defining Limits

Knowing yourself means being able to sense when you have hit the anaerobic threshold; that is, when you're exhausting your energy reserves at a rate faster than you can replenish them. A good sign that you're pushing the limit is when your legs start to burn—but by then it's a bit late. Do more than a few seconds of anaerobic work, and you've cut into your overall performance for the day. Often this will happen on a hill, but it can also happen when your ego makes you chase a more experienced rider on flat terrain.

As Paul Jurbala, a Canadian exercise physiologist, explained, "Crossing the anaerobic threshold is accompanied by a sudden increase in the depth and rate of breathing. At one point you will be working fairly hard, and be breathing deeply; work a little harder, and your breathing will seem to increase by a disproportionate amount. This, very roughly, will be your anaerobic threshold."

Racers train to improve their anaerobic threshold by riding a strenuous interval workout at least once a week. If you're really ambitious, you may want to do this during one or two of your mid-week training rides, as it will indeed strengthen you for hills, head winds, and catching up with friends. But don't train that way on your long-distance days. If you are breathing hard and your sweat glands are gushing, shift down, slow down, and enjoy a more relaxed pace. Twirl the pedals and avoid the feeling that your feet are pushing heavy weights. Remember, you're going after a personal distance record. There will be

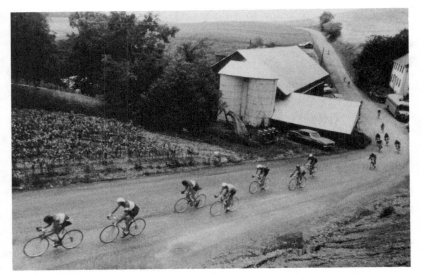

Photograph 3–3. On your first century ride, don't try to compete with anyone else. Just ride your own pace and rest assured you will see some of the early speedsters again before the day is over.

plenty of time later to build big, hill-smashing quadriceps—especially if you manage to preserve your knees today.

Even if you disregard this advice for part of the ride, it is never too late to retreat to the spinning mode. A few pieces of fruit and a shift to lower gears for the final miles have brought many a would-be centurian happily to the finish. It also helps to have an odometer to occasionally check against the elapsed time. If you did 80 miles in 8 hours, you can aim for 100 miles in 10 hours. If you leave the 25-mile rest stop/checkpoint 2½ hours after the start, that is about right for a 10-hour century. But evaluate the conditions for the day and route. Hills, head winds, or extreme heat should make you set your pace a notch or two lower.

Here are some more basic rules to observe when riding centuries.

- Never force the pace, especially during the early hours of riding.
- Never ride until you are so exhausted you cannot eat or rest.
- Keep your rests short and infrequent to maintain your rhythm.

Long breaks are fun for socializing, but they will ruin your pace, and you will have to "warm-up" your muscles all over again. Aim for a 30- to 45-minute rest. Get in, eat, greet your friends, relax a few minutes, relieve yourself, stretch some, and return to the road.

Food for Fuel

The rule of thumb for century riders is to "eat before you're hungry and drink before you're thirsty." It's good advice. You are not likely to overeat or drink during a ride, but you do need to avoid indulging in the wrong foods. Walter Ezell discovered that pizza and iced tea were a bad combination on his first ride. Use your common sense and experience in choosing the type of food that will work well for you.

As you begin to ride longer distances, your eating habits must change. The muscles and liver can store enough glycogen for you to ride hard for several hours—especially if your diet for the preceding day was high in carbohydrates. But to complete a century ride, even at a relaxed pace, you have to eat along the way. Part of your training, as we said before, is to notice how your body reacts to various types of foods. Fortunately, you don't have to worry about counting the number of calories you consume since a 150-pound person will probably burn more than 5,000 calories while riding a century.

For a pre-event meal, experts recommend a diet high in complex carbohydrates (starchy foods such as pasta, bread, potatoes, and rice), low in fat, and low in protein. Fat has twice as many calories per gram as carbohydrates and protein, but it is harder to digest and slows the digestion of other foods as well. It is true that participants in the cross-continent Great American Bike Race craved fatty foods, but then these were ultra-endurance athletes who were living on their bikes for days on end! Research done by William Evans of Tufts University indicates that endurance athletes can train their bodies to burn fat more efficiently than ordinary people and thus gain an important source of energy.

However, a century ride is far from a ride across the continent, so you would be well advised to stick with carbohydrates for ease of digestion and a readily available source of energy.

Carbohydrates found in fresh fruits, for example, will give you needed fuel for pedaling. At the same time, fruit contains minerals and some of the water you need to replenish what is lost through perspiration. By eating enough of the right foods, you avoid what some cyclists call "the bonk," the go-no-more feeling you get when your body runs out of fuel. If this ever happens to you, the combination of rest and a few pieces of fresh fruit or fruit juice can work wonders.

Stories are told of cyclists who set out on a century ride without food in hopes of losing weight, only to end up pushing their bikes home. Don't try to fast on a century! If, in fact, you arrive home from a century and find you are five pounds lighter, congratulations are not in order. Almost all of that five pounds lost will undoubtedly be water. You should have drunk more fluids. And do not wait until you feel thirsty; make yourself drink. A good rule of thumb is to consume one pint of water every hour, particularly on very hot days. Quantities will vary with the temperature, your pace, conditioning, and body weight. Your training rides will teach you to gauge how much water you need to drink. In addition, cool water poured on you is a good way to beat the heat.

A Little Goes a Long Way

It is unlikely that you'll overtrain, but you should recognize the signs. A mild illness, a joint or muscle injury, or constant fatigue can mean you're doing too much, too fast. Keep in mind that the way an athlete becomes stronger is to stress the muscles (including the heart) and then allow them to recover. Stress, recover, stress, recover—that's the pattern.

One way to prevent overtraining and monitor your progress is to start a training diary. By keeping a daily log of your mileage, pace, and how your body responds to training (including your resting pulse rate in the morning), it's a good bet you won't go off the deep end.

But if you do overdo it, here's the advice Tom Moore of the Niagara Frontier Bicycle Club once gave:

"Take two or three days off from riding and see a good movie. When you start again, drop your weekly mileage to what it was two or three weeks before, and make your weekly increases smaller."

Keep the Pace

Racers and tourists-in-a-hurry often ride single file close behind each other to take advantage of decreased wind resistance. This is known as riding in a paceline. On your first century, you probably should not attempt to join a paceline. All it takes is a moment of weary inattention, two wheels touch, and the following rider crashes—along with any who are behind him.

Riding in pace is an important skill for racers, and it can be exhilarating when everyone in the line knows the necessary precautions and procedures. But if you train shorter distances without a paceline, you can complete a century without a paceline.

The Essentials

Don't show up at the starting line with a lot of newly purchased and untested gear. Start your ride with equipment that is broken in, road tested, and comfortable. Bring along a helmet, one or two water bottles, a comfortable saddle, a well-

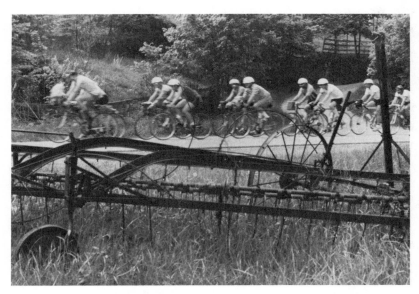

Photograph 3–4. Experienced riders often ride in lines close behind one another to decrease wind resistance. Because of the danger of crashing, don't try to learn paceline riding on your first century.

adjusted and lubricated bike you're used to, gearing appropriate for the terrain, tools, patch kit, spare tube, pump, food, money, and a first aid kit.

We also recommend touring shoes, cycling shorts (worn without underwear), cycling gloves, a small handlebar bag (don't overload it), rain cape and fenders (if rain is likely), windbreaker, compass, map, and odometer. Many club rides furnish cue sheets for navigating the route ("3.2 miles, right on Ferngate Rd."), so an odometer is valuable for anticipating turns.

Century Training at a Glance

If you have a full-time job and family, you won't have time for long workouts on weekdays. On these days, ride about 45 minutes at a pace strenuous enough to strengthen your muscles and work your heart. Then on Saturdays and Sundays aim for distance, keeping in mind the stress-recovery pattern discussed earlier.

If you are a beginner, start your training program with your current best distance and increase that by 25 to 30 percent every Saturday. Keep a relaxed, steady pace. On Sunday, cut your Saturday mileage in half, again concentrating on pace and position on the bike. During weekdays, stick with shorter, more strenuous rides, introducing some hills as the weeks progress.

Here is a sample, two-month schedule for beginning riders.

Weeks 1 to 2: Are you still introducing yourself to the bike? Now is the time to perfect gearing and braking techniques. Concentrate on pedaling steadily without interruption. On weekdays, go for short rides, every day if possible. Increase your daily mileage slowly, no more than 1 to 3 miles a day. On your first Saturday, ride 12 miles at a steady pace. On Sunday, ride 6 miles. The following week, ride 17 miles on Saturday, dropping back to 8 miles on Sunday.

Weeks 3 to 4: You can step up the regimen slightly, including rolling terrain on some of your weekday rides and increasing your weekend mileage. The emphasis now is on technique and distance. Pay close attention to your position and riding technique to develop good riding habits. This is the time to modify your position if you need to, not the night before a century. On your third Saturday, ride 25 miles. That Sunday, ride 12. On the fourth Saturday of training, aim to ride 32 miles, dropping back on Sunday to 16 miles. (At this point, what seemed to be a hard distance three weeks earlier is now your "easy" day.)

Weeks 5 to 6: You should now concentrate on pace. Your daily rides should leave you tired but not exhausted. You can try to push your speed a bit during these shorter rides since by occasionally overloading the muscles you can train them to recover quickly, thereby increasing your power on the hills and speed on the flats. At the same time, approach your weekend rides as dress rehearsal centuries. On your fifth Saturday, ride 40 miles, cutting down to 20 miles on Sunday. The following week, ride 50 miles on Saturday and 25 on Sunday.

Weeks 7 to 8: During the seventh week, you may want to experiment with your training a bit. You can pepper your daily training rides with a few short intervals. For example, after you've warmed up, pick a point like a hilltop, signpost, or road marker several hundred yards ahead and go for it as hard as you can. That Saturday, ride 65 miles, followed by a 32-miler on Sunday. By the eighth and final week, you'll be riding your farthest—so you may want to relax the pace a bit on your weekday rides. Ride 80 miles on Saturday, followed by a 40-miler on Sunday.

Week 9: Don't stay away from the bike, but don't push too hard. Thursday, take a short ride to loosen your muscles. On Saturday, you complete your century and earn your patch. Now visit the friends and relatives who think you've all but disappeared.

Embracing the Discipline of the Double

When giving advice concerning the double century, we start with the assumption that you are already able to ride a century in a fair amount of comfort. Otherwise, it makes no sense for you to be training to ride twice that distance. The training schedule that we recommend for this event really picks up where the one for a century leaves off. That means your longer training rides are now 70 to 85 miles and that you can ride 100 miles on any given weekend in six to seven hours.

As is true for the century, the ultimate goal in your double-century training program is absolute familiarity with yourself on the bicycle both physically and emotionally. What is the best pace for you? What foods should you eat and in what quantities? How do you feel after riding 140 miles? How do you relieve boredom or depression late in a double century? Successful double-century rides depend a lot on this type of self-knowledge.

Physically, you need to spend a lot of time on the bike. Even though you may be now riding a few hundred miles per week in 30- to 40-mile increments, there is no substitute for putting in long miles in one session. Whereas your longest rides for centuries were 80 miles, you will now be extending your mileage into the 120- to 150-mile range. Inevitably, your workout schedule will occasionally take a back seat to family and career; in these instances, you can substitute shorter, more intense training rides. These training sessions will help you become familiar with the gearing, pace, and riding position that you can maintain in comfort for long hours.

As with the century, the double should not be approached as a race. Be especially wary of getting caught up in the frenzy of the start, which is more a release of tension than a rational decision to ride fast. And watch out both for undisciplined beginners and seasoned racers. The former won't understand pacing, and the latter simply have you outclassed. Trying to maintain the early pace of either one will negate your own well-planned strategy. Instead, relax, let them go, and be secure in the thought that you'll see most of them again before the ride is over.

Proper Diet

An important part of successfully completing a double century comes from learning how to pace yourself with food and drink. In a century, you can get by with eating once, say at the halfway point, and still survive. In a double, however, it is essential to start eating before the 80- to 90-mile mark so you'll feel well nourished and fresh to ride another 100 or so miles.

Perhaps a more subtle aspect of the double century is the greater need for a variety of snack foods. You'll get awfully bored with eating bananas or granola bars for 14 hours straight. Use your longer training rides to experiment with various types of food and feeding schedules. Among the more popular are granola bars, peanut butter and jelly sandwiches, sliced fruit, raisins, nuts, and bananas. Your diet off the bike should be well balanced, including foods from the four basic food groups. There's no need to start making drastic changes in your daily diet, just be sure you're eating good meals on a regular basis.

During the ride, remember to drink before you're thirsty and eat before you're hungry. An enormous amount of fluid loss occurs during a ride of this length, and most riders fail to recognize how fast it is happening. A good rule of thumb is to consume one pint-size water bottle of fluid for every hour on the road. Many double-century riders prefer carrying one bottle of an electrolyte replacement fluid for drinking and one bottle of water for dousing themselves. Others, like Andy Schafer, an experienced double-century rider from California, prefer to drink only water between rest stops. Use your training rides to determine which fluids and in what quantities work best for you.

You can expect to burn between 8,000 and 12,000 calories in the course of those 200 miles. It is virtually impossible to eat enough calories during the event to match that energy output, but you can buffer yourself against problems by eating a high-carbohydrate meal with foods like pasta, rice, or potatoes the night before. Then, during the event, your eating pattern should be one of nonstop nibbling, what Schafer calls a "progressive snack." Using this technique, you should be able to eat an additional 4,000 to 6,000 calories.

The idea is to eat in small amounts continuously so that you never overload the digestive system but maintain a steady flow of fresh energy to the muscles. The natural lag time between ingestion of food and its availability to provide energy dictates that you eat early and frequently in the event in order to constantly replenish the bloodstream with glucose, a carbohydrate derivative. If you wait until you begin feeling hungry and try to compensate by eating a copious meal, all you will get is a full gut.

Schafer recommends that first-time double-century riders take advantage of the food provided by the sponsor at every

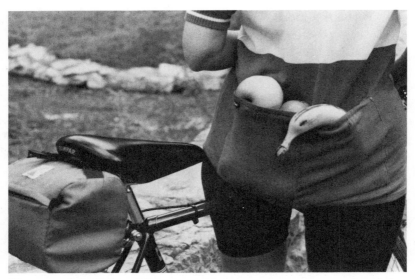

Photograph 3–5. In addition to eating a good pre-race meal and the fare offered at rest stops, you may want to carry along some fresh fruit for pedaling fuel and replacement of water lost through perspiration.

rest stop, saving personal pocket food for times between stops. The length of these stops will vary with the weather conditions and your own personal requirements. During hotter days, take a little longer to cool down; on cooler days, it will be to your advantage to keep the rest stops shorter. In all cases, particularly for the lunch stop, try to eat right away, then relax for a bit, stretch, give your body a chance to digest some of the food.

Enduring to the End

The later stages of the double are perhaps the most challenging, both physically and psychologically. Besides the onset of physical fatigue, those last few miles can be characterized by temporary bouts of depression, a sort of psychological no-man's land where the rider can begin to lose enthusiasm for the ride. Again, have the discipline to listen to what your body and mind are telling you and respond accordingly. If the pace has become laborious and difficult to maintain, gear down and spin for a while. Try to relax, eat a piece of fruit, and enjoy yourself. Within a few minutes, you will find yourself picking up the pace again because your level of exertion has fallen below what causes you discomfort.

If that doesn't do the trick, try getting off the bike for five minutes or so. Taking those few minutes to stretch, use the bathroom, or just move around a bit will make a tremendous difference in your enjoyment of the final miles. The important idea here is not to be afraid to reward yourself in whatever physical or psychological ways you can to guarantee a successful finish. And give yourself a pat on the back when you do!

Double-Century Training at a Glance

Since most cyclists have both a family and career, training for a double century often takes the form of long, intense weekend rides, supplemented during the week with shorter speed workouts and commutes to work. To follow this weekly schedule, you must be reasonably fit—able to ride 75 to 80 miles at a time comfortably.

Weeks 1 to 3: The first few weeks should be spent getting your comfortable mileage over the 100-mile mark. Extend the mileage of your rides no more than 15 percent at a time. Do an 80-mile ride the first week, 90 plus the next, and perhaps 110 the following week. If you do this long ride on Saturday, take an easier ride on Sunday, no more than 40 or 50 miles, concentrating on form and cadence. During the week, you should continue your shorter, higher intensity rides, alternating between spinning and higher-geared speed work.

Because your rides will be starting earlier or ending later, you will be able to start experimenting with wearing and carrying different types of cycling clothing. There will be times when you'll need leg warmers or tights for an early morning start but then need to remove them for the remainder of the day. Similarly, some of the mountainous areas where double centuries are often staged can undergo rapid changes in weather. In that case, how do you carry a Gore-Tex jacket or other appropriate rain gear? You should think not only about types of clothing necessary but also efficient ways to attach them to your bicycle. Also, begin experimenting with different foods to eat while riding, trying to expand your repertoire.

Weeks 4 to 5: Now we begin the more important psychological training. The big change in your rides will be intensity. Continue to ride 100 to 120 miles at a brisk pace on Saturday. On Sunday of the fourth week, ride 50 to 60 miles, but again, at a high level of exertion. The fifth week, extend that Sunday distance to 75 to 80 miles. The short overnight resting period will begin to help simulate the rigors of the double. Knowing that you can go hard, then go hard soon again, will also begin to strengthen both your mental and physical reserves.

Weeks 6 to 9: For the final four weeks preceding the double, you should ride, as a minimum, over 100 miles at a high exertion

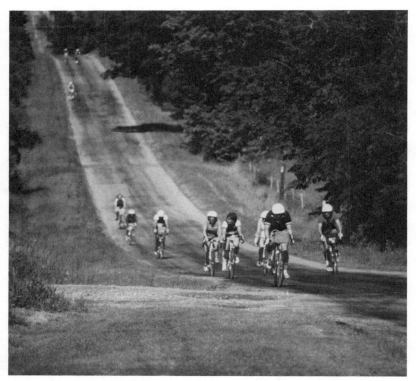

Photograph 3–6. Climbing hills can be especially tough late in a double century ride, so it is a good idea to include interval hill training among your regular workouts.

level on both Saturday and Sunday. If possible, try to extend one of these rides into the 120- to 150-mile range. Your time goal for your first double ought to be 14 to 16 hours. So, if you are riding back-to-back centuries, try to ride Saturday's century in 6 to 7 hours, with Sunday's ride no slower than 7 to 8 hours. Again, it is as much a psychological exercise as it is a physical one.

Don't be afraid to mix up the training tempos a little bit. Even though the emphasis is on distance and rhythm, high-cadence spinning and interval speed training are still essential for maintaining quickness in your legs, what the racers commonly refer to as "snap."

Andy Schafer, whose best double-century time is 10 hours, 20 minutes, recommends combining interval hill training with longer rides to improve endurance. "As you approach a hill during your workout, attack it," he says. "Then, see how fast you recuperate. As you get into better condition, your recuperation period will become very, very short." At the top of the hill, Schafer recommends, relax, spin a little, take a drink, and before you know it, you'll be ready to continue again at a very strong pace. Besides improving your physical condition, he claims, this interval training also gives you the confidence of knowing you've got a little extra reserve of energy to draw on late in a double century.

Maintenance and Repair

There is a price to pay, of course, for all these training miles. While your body has been getting fitter and fitter, your clothing and equipment have been undergoing their share of wear and tear. Taking time to ensure that such things as shoe cleats, cycling shorts, and jerseys are in good repair could prevent an unpleasant surprise on the day of the event.

Also, the week before the double (not the night before) you should replace both front and rear tires on your bike. There's no point in going through ten weeks of dedicated training for the double century, only to have tire fatigue destroy an otherwise successful effort.

It's also important during this last week to get plenty of sleep and eat well-balanced meals. You are building a foundation for success on the weekend. By Friday or Saturday night, you may be too wound up to rest properly. Your cycling during this final week should be a little more relaxed. If possible, try to do several 50- to 70-milers.

The day before the event, take one final ride, no more than 25 or 30 easy miles, as a final test ride of your equipment. Any bike maintenance should be limited to ensuring that all bolts and screws are tight, that your spare tire and handlebar bag are securely fastened, and that your water bottles are full. You might want to go through the racer's exercise of cleaning your bicycle top to bottom. Besides ensuring that your bike is in top working order, it helps put you in a confident frame of mind, knowing that you have done all the training and that your mind, body, and bicycle are ready.

Finally, eat an early dinner and go to bed. Tomorrow you will open the door to a whole new world of cycling adventures.

Part Four
Super-Fitness through Multisport Training

Total Fitness through Cross-Training

Philosophies of athletic training are no less a matter of debate than the ideas that underlie other disciplines. There is no one path to religious or moral understanding. Physicists cannot agree on the structure of the atom or the origin of the universe. So it is not surprising that when it comes to maintenance of the human body, the most complex of organisms, a wide range of opinions exist.

A bedrock rule in modern athletics is the principle of specificity of training: if you are going to compete in 25-mile time trials, you had better ride lots of them. If you want to be good at velodrome sprint events, spend your time practicing those skills. There's little value in a cyclist (to exaggerate the point) practicing hundreds of free throws on the basketball court.

But an athletic development of the 1980s calls for some reconsideration of this principle. Many amateur athletes in this decade are no longer interested in simply riding a club century or running a 10K race. They find multisport events more interesting and challenging. The most popular and best known events are triathlons—combinations of swimming, bicycling, and running. In 1983, *Triathlon* magazine estimated that 100,000 athletes would participate in triathlons that year alone. And the number seems to be growing steadily.

In nearly every case, these *triathletes* are people who previously thought of themselves as basically runners, cyclists, or swimmers. To prepare for a triathlon, they had to switch from single event training to training for three different events at the same time.

What these athletes sometimes report is that crossover or synergistic effects come into play from this kind of "cross-training." Long miles of running, for instance, can yield a level of cardiovascular fitness that improves bicycling or swimming performances.

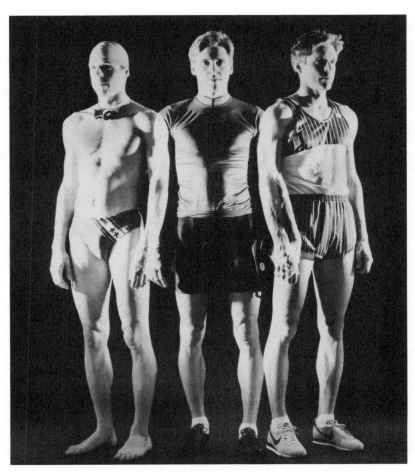

Photograph 4–1. Multisport training and competition has become quite popular in recent years. Many athletes find it mentally refreshing and physically more beneficial than concentrating on a single sport.

But there are benefits to be derived from cross-training that have relevance for every athlete, even those who never intend to compete in more than one sport or those uninterested in formal competition at all. By engaging in a variety of forms of exercise you can (1) avoid boredom or "burn-out" from doing too much of one thing, (2) avoid injuries from overuse and reduce lost time from those that do occur, (3) improve your overall fitness level, and (4) maintain your conditioning throughout all seasons and all types of weather.

A Mental Refresher

Canadian coach Norman Sheil, who trained national cycling teams for 18 years, believes that rest is as important a part of an athlete's program as are the details of the workout. For Sheil, part of rest is "getting away from it all," including using free time for an activity that has nothing to do with bicycles. "When I was racing in Europe, a lot of us would go fishing. That's really getting away from it all, but having that different activity kept me fresh and eager."

Sheil is speaking, of course, of the kind of athlete who spends an entire day riding, doing weight workouts, and then more riding. For such an athlete, physical exhaustion coupled with mental burn-out can be a real problem. As a cyclist, you probably do not spend nearly so much time in the saddle as these top athletes, but you also don't have a coach to tell you when to vary your activities.

So what are the signs that might indicate you need a break? Ed Burke, technical director of the United States Cycling Federation, says that all kinds of riders are susceptible to an occasional letdown: "You are not fired up for the ride ahead of you. You're lethargic. You feel tired all the time, or you're tired before you even start a ride. You may discover that your heart rate is elevated a bit."

Burke says it's long been recognized that attitude can affect the efficiency of training, so it makes good sense for recreational riders to be aware that they can overdo it when building up their mileage in preparation for a century. By adding a day of running or replacing a ride with a weight-lifting session, for

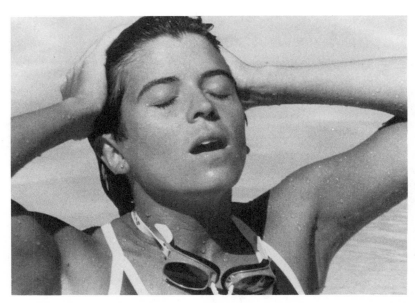

Photograph 4–2. Swimming is the best aerobic exercise for developing the upper body and is the first event in a triathlon.

instance, your weekly schedule can be varied enough so that you can prevent a slump. Besides, by substituting an activity instead of just taking a day off, even very conscientious riders need not feel guilty about this time off the bicycle.

Rx for Overuse

Injuries from overuse are not common among recreational cyclists, but they do happen. According to Burke, tendinitis and aching knees are two of the most frequent complaints. However, it's far more likely for a runner to turn to bicycling because his 40 miles a week have taken their toll. Runners suffering from knee trouble, stress fractures, and back trouble report that after getting clearance from a doctor, their aches "go away" when they switch to riding a bicycle, with little or no loss in cardio-vascular fitness.

If you like both running and riding, another way to apply this principle is to decrease your mileage of one while adding

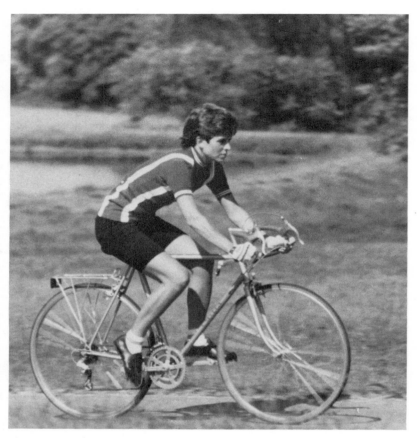

Photograph 4–3. Many runners who develop overuse injuries turn to cycling as an alternative. Cycling is the middle event in a triathlon.

to the other. Your total workout time doesn't have to change, and by cutting back, overuse injuries can be avoided before they happen. Dr. George Sheehan, M.D., who frequently writes and lectures on the subject of running, suggests that 25 miles weekly seems to be the level at which injuries start to crop up among runners. By limiting your running and supplementing with cycling in a few training sessions, you can still spend the same "quality" time working out, injury free.

Peter Van Handle, an exercise physiologist who works with the United States Olympic Committee (USOC), says an examination of how muscles function shows the way cross-training comes into play in the conditioning of the legs. During an activity like sprinting on the bicycle, the rider's nervous system activates the muscle cells needed for the task. While riding, this repeated recruitment of muscle cells in the quadriceps, for example, builds up that muscle.

"But in running, you are relying on different muscle cells, including the hamstrings and those in the shins," he says. Muscles operate in pairs, with agonists starting a motion (like the quadriceps moving the leg up and forward) and antagonists returning the motion (like the hamstrings). If only half of the pair is well developed, the half that has to resist its motion can be strained. So, when both the front and back of the leg are exercised in a sensible program of cross-training, overuse injuries, such as tendinitis and ligament strain, are less likely to occur.

Cardiovascular Conditioning

There are advantages to multisport training, including the benefits derived from regular aerobic workouts to strengthen the lungs and circulatory system. But there's no guarantee that just because you're a powerful swimmer you'll necessarily be a first-rate cyclist immediately, if ever. "In swimming, you primarily use the arms," Ed Burke points out, "and in cycling you rely on the legs. Becoming adept at several sports means building up your muscles through training over time. But you will derive the benefits of greater cardiovascular fitness right away."

Burke suggests, though, that two factors make it hard to generalize about just how much payback each person can expect. First is the matter of skill and technique. If you are swimming with a clean, economical stroke, minute-for-minute or lap-for-lap, you can derive more training benefits from the sport than someone who splashes around like a panicky dog. Or, consider the relative amount of work done by a rider who knows how to use his gears and one who doesn't. The skilled cyclist will be able to ride at the pace required to elevate his or her heart rate and strengthen the cardiovascular system. An adept cyclist can also stave off the fatigue that a beginner, who's still struggling to find the right gears, often feels in a training session.

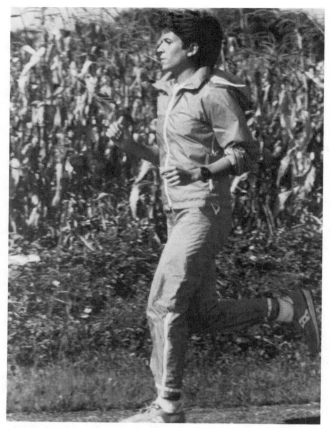

Photograph 4–4. Running remains one of the most popular ways to develop cardiovascular conditioning, and a long-distance race forms the final event in a triathlon.

Burke says that because of these variables, there is no common denominator that will allow him to say how an hour of riding compares to running or swimming.

There also is the factor of individual differences among athletes. Someone who has the determination to work at a certain level of effort will become fitter than one who doesn't. "How hard can you push yourself? If you can work your heart at a rate of 160 to 180 beats per minute for 20 minutes or so, you will be more fit than someone who pushes to that level and then backs off," Burke says.

Off-Season Efforts

Experts insistent on sport-specific training during the competitive season usually acknowledge the value of cross-training during other times of the year. Well-known examples of people who have successfully engaged in seasonal alternations between sports are Eric and Beth Heiden. They gained national fame as speed skaters at the 1980 Winter Olympics. For off-season work, they rode bicycles, and it turned out they were pretty good at that, too. (Eric has since turned pro on the bike, and Beth won the women's world championship road race in 1980.)

Canada's Sheil says with a bit of understatement that Canadians "don't have the pleasure of doing much riding in the winter." So, he recommends cross-country skiing or weight training as money in the bank that will pay its dividends in the following bicycling season. Speed skating emphasizes almost the same muscles as bicycling. But, Sheil says, suitable speed skating rinks are pretty hard to find, even in Canada.

Burke says, "I can ride a bike. I can run or go skiing. I'm just keeping in shape. For that level of fitness, cross-training is valuable." Add to that the important factor of attitude. Stan Lindstedt, a bicyclist as well as a muscle physiologist at the University of Wyoming, points out that while research in cross-training is just beginning, many cyclists know what works for them based on personal experience. "If I go running and feel that because of bicycling, my running on the hills has improved, then who cares what the laboratory says anyway?"

So whether you are a budding triathlete or just an ordinary person interested in getting in top physical and mental condition, cross-training has much to offer you. It will inject welcome variety into your daily activities, strengthen all parts of your body and your cardiovascular system while minimizing the chance of muscle injury, and provide a way for you to keep fit and trim 12 months of every year.

Why and How to Cross-Train

A strange twist of fate led Jennifer Hinshaw into triathlon competition. At age 16, she was a nationally ranked swimmer with Olympic potential, but an automobile accident in which she broke her neck put an end to thoughts of swimming competitively. After recuperating from the injury, Jennifer resumed recreational swimming but lost her ambition to return to the six hour a day training she had previously pursued and began to look elsewhere for challenges.

In 1982, Jennifer's family convinced her to take up bike riding. On her first day out, her younger brother led her up the meanest, steepest hills he could find. One of them was a two-mile climb where the grade gets as steep as 15 percent. Though she complained at the time, she later realized that having survived that climb she could tackle anything. A month after that initial ride, she was training in earnest for the Hawaii Ironman Triathlon. After only three months of training, she finished ninth among the women at the 1982 Ironman. She came away from her first triathlon more determined than ever and increased her training mileage substantially in preparation for the 1983 Ironman.

Jennifer sees advantages and disadvantages in multisport training. "If you want to be the very best in a sport such as swimming, running, or cycling, then you've got to devote yourself to that activity exclusively. But if you're looking for sport as recreation, then a varied training program is a good idea. Mastering running, cycling, and swimming doesn't necessarily mean you have to compete in a triathlon either—you may just like the feeling of overall fitness."

Looking back on her previous experience as a competitive swimmer, Jennifer comments: "A variety of sports makes training more interesting. Swimming six hours a day was monotonous—I don't think I'll ever train solely for one sport again." Though she is no longer as good a swimmer as she was when she trained only for swimming, she feels that cross-training has made her stronger. "Swimming exercises your upper arms and gives you overall fitness. Running develops the lower body. And cycling not only gives me leg strength but lung power as well."

Carol Hogan is a woman in her late forties. A few years ago,

Carol and her husband, active members in a cycling club, decided to ride their bikes across the country. To prepare for the effort, Carol spent months cycling, lifting weights, and running. In the process, she discovered that she enjoyed the challenge of tackling several sports at once. She was also inspired by the sight of John Howard stepping across the finish line at the 1981 Hawaii Ironman Triathlon.

After completing her cross-country bike ride, Carol Hogan decided to train for the 1982 Ironman. An interview with John Howard had given her a pretty good idea of the kind of training she had to do. Six months later, she competed in the triathlon and finished third in her age group (45 to 49).

Carol has managed to balance involvement in sports with pursuit of a career as a photojournalist. Fortunately, her husband shares her interest in athletics since the combined pressures of career, family, and triathlon training are quite intense. The remainder of this chapter is based on suggestions that Carol offers to those interested in multisport training.

Getting Started

First of all, it is good to remember that you don't have to be interested in competing in a triathlon like the Hawaii Ironman or even one of the mini-triathlons currently being staged in various parts of the country to find cross-training worthwhile. You can use it, as Jennifer also suggested, to gain and maintain overall fitness, or you can use it to help prevent overuse injuries in one sport that you wish to pursue competitively. Whatever your purpose is for cross-training, it helps to get it clear in your mind before you begin because it will affect the amount of time and level of effort you need to put into it. Also, consider the effect of your training on your family, your career, and the other activities in life you find worthwhile.

A good way to approach your decision about your goals is to sit down and work out a schedule. Begin by calculating how much free time you really have to train. It's amazing how many hours are spent on the job, as well as commuting, running errands, and keeping up with personal and home maintenance.

Be realistic—if you can spare only an hour or two each day, don't dream about being number one in the Ironman.

If you're considering competition, you will have to cope with a great deal of mental pressure about how to spend your time. Carol Hogan found that when she was out seriously training, she worried whether she should be at her job, and when she was working at her job, she kept thinking about the long bike rides she should be taking. She also found that the best way to balance training with family is to include them in the training as much as possible. You can run in a park they can enjoy, with a picnic after; spend the day at the beach (or pool) where you can swim; employ spouse and children to act as timers, to research training information, or to serve as bike handlers in races. Drawing them into the circle instead of leaving them out will only increase their support.

A Few Training Tips

Once you have clearly assessed your available time and decided on your goals, you should map out a basic training program. If this program is going to involve a substantial increase in the level of activity to which you are accustomed or if you are over 40 years of age, consult your physician. Tell him what you have in mind and have him give you a thorough examination. If he gives you the green light, you are ready to start training.

To be a top-notch triathlete, you should work out every day, but not everyone can afford that luxury. The beauty of multisport training is that it offers flexibility; you can work at your own pace and level of fitness. The only guideline is to exercise three or four times a week to strengthen your cardiovascular system.

If you're already accomplished in one sport, such as cycling, the best approach is to train at a maintenance level in that one and to work harder on the others. Also, every day devoted to training should consist of primary and supplemental workouts. The reason? To benefit from multisport training, you must stress yourself one sport at a time. Some athletes make the mistake of trying to train in every sport equally each day. But if you do that, you'll quickly reach a plateau with little chance of improvement. Instead, devote one day primarily to swimming, one to running, one to cycling.

On your swimming day, plan on spending at least two hours in the water doing a series of intervals to develop strength and stamina. Then take a short bike ride and a run. On another day, focus on running for your primary workout and supplement your exercise routine with a brief swim and bike ride and so on.

Start out with a training load in each activity that is appropriate for your current level of fitness. Plan small but regular increments in distance, particularly with running, if that aspect of the training is new to you. Running too far too soon is an invitation to overuse injury. It takes time for your joints to accustom themselves to the pounding of the sport. Many an enthusiastic runner has moved rapidly into high mileage only to incur an injury that set his training back for weeks. So easy does it at the start.

If possible, do some of your training in the morning or at noon and some in late afternoon or evening to reduce the chances of a physical "overload" and to give your routine some variety. You don't have to train for all three sports at the same time of day; though if you're training for triathlons, you need to include some workouts in which you experience swim-to-bike and bike-to-run transitions to see how they feel.

Whether your training schedule is your own creation or one you obtain from a more seasoned athlete, never forget that it is only an aid, not an inflexible guide. There will be times when you must and should deviate from it. Sure, some days you will start out feeling tired, then your energy and enthusiasm will return once your workout is underway. But, if you begin to feel tired all the time, your legs always heavy as lead, and you find yourself dreading every workout, it is time to take a day off.

If you intend to work out six or seven days a week, schedule in an alternation between hard days and easy days. Otherwise, your body will not have enough chance to recuperate from the stress it is experiencing, your performance will become consistently sluggish, and you will begin to burn out on the whole enterprise. So schedule your workouts wisely and become sensitive enough to your body to know when and how to depart from that schedule.

Getting into Swimming

How much you should swim depends a great deal on your age and ability. A general rule of thumb is to start with a distance with which you feel comfortable and gradually increase it. Your level of endurance will definitely increase with practice.

Since swimming technique is difficult to learn from a book, you may require coaching. Carol Hogan took a course to improve the mechanics of her stroke. In this course, she learned ways to improve her speed and alleviate boredom and was started on a weight-training program to strengthen her swimming muscles. A call to your local Department of Parks and Recreation, gymnasium, health club, or Y may turn up a class of this sort. Also, many school pools throughout the country open their doors to masters swimming groups and recreational swimming on evenings and weekends.

A pool is the place to work on perfecting stroke technique and increasing both your speed and stamina. With the aid of a timer, find out what pace per 100 meters you can hold for 500 meters. Work on holding that pace for 800, then 1,000, and on up to 1,500 meters and more. After that, work on quickening your pace as you again move from shorter to longer distances. As with everything else, the speed at which you should attempt to progress in this program depends on your goal; a triathlete will probably push herself harder over the weeks than someone multitraining for recreation.

Whatever your training goals, eventually you'll want to do intervals—swimming sets such as 5 × 100 meters, 10 × 100 meters, and so on—with specific rest periods ranging from 10 to 30 seconds between each 100 meters. Intervals build strength and endurance and add variety to your routine.

If you are preparing for a triathlon, open water swimming—lake or ocean, depending on where your event will be held—is also essential. You need to accustom yourself to the motion of waves and learn to swim a straight line without the benefit of pool lane stripes. If you don't swim regularly in open water

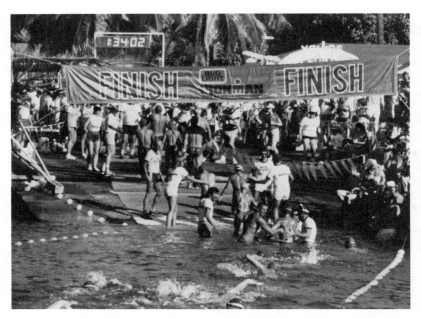

Photograph 4–5. The swim finish at the 1983 Hawaii Ironman
Triathlon.

before your event, it's too easy to panic in sudden awareness
that the water is very deep and the lake or ocean shore is far
away!

When you swim in an ocean or lake, you need to take
special precautions. Carol Hogan experienced several close en-
counters with trolling lines, barge propellers, and the like. She
soon began wearing a bright orange swimming cap and avoided
the open water except for organized events. No matter where
you swim, it's important to warm up before going at it vigorously. At the start, you feel so fresh that it's easy to go out too
hard and fast. Then you quickly feel out of breath and tired. To
prevent that, warm up with long, steady strokes at an unhurried
pace.

A Swim Worksheet

Newcomers to swimming often underestimate the rigors
of the sport. It's important to remember that when you swim,
particularly in a lake or ocean, *don't overextend.* Be sure you
have enough energy to get back to shore.

Here is a sample weekly workout program to start you off.

Sunday: Swim in the ocean for a specific length of time—a half hour is good—using a variety of strokes. You'll find spending time in the salty deep with waves that constantly knock you around tiring, so it's all right to tread water. The idea at first is simply to accustom yourself to swimming in rough water. Over the weeks, you can use landmarks such as a buoy, water tower, or lighthouse to keep track of your distance.

Monday: Your first day in a pool should start with warming up by swimming at a comfortable pace for 200 to 300 yards (12 laps in a 25-yard pool). Bring or borrow a kickboard and exercise your legs by kicking vigorously for 100 yards. Use a pull buoy (a triangular piece of polystyrene that fits between your legs and comes with two hand-held ropes) so you can "pull" yourself along, concentrating on stroke technique and building up the upper body. Then do a "cool-down" of continuous laps for 200 to 300 yards at a comfortable pace.

Tuesday: No swimming.

Wednesday: Repeat of Monday's routine. You can try intervals, swimming 50 yards and using a timer (available at some pools) or your own wristwatch to keep track of your pace. Repeat a routine of swimming hard for 50 yards—taking a 10- to 30-second rest break—and swimming again for as many times as you can, usually no more than five times for a novice. (Longer rest breaks may be appealing but won't help you stress yourself.)

Thursday: No swimming.

Friday: Follow a similar pool routine with a warm-up, kicking, pulling, intervals (in 50-yard increments), and a cool-down. Your routine doesn't have to be in this order as long as you always start with a warm-up and end with a cool-down session.

Saturday: This is an "easy swim" day in which you concentrate more on your stroke than speed or distance.

Tackling the Open Road

The best place to get involved in cycling is at a reputable bike shop, which offers knowledgeable salespeople and a good selection of frames. They'll also know of any racing or recreational clubs in the local area. You don't need top-of-the-line equipment to start. Many very good bicycles are available in

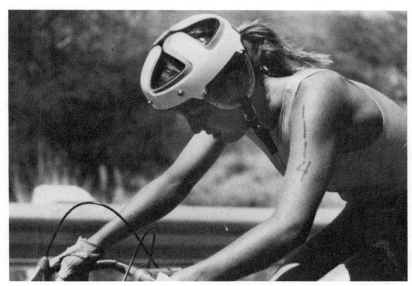

Photograph 4–6. Patricia Puntous, second place woman finisher at the '83 Ironman, riding in the cycling event.

the $300 to 400 range so keep your budget in mind when buying new equipment.

One piece of equipment that's critical to your riding is a helmet. Don't leave the bike shop without one! All races require them; many triathlons now only accept the hard-shell type. But even if you never set wheel in a race, your helmet can protect you from serious injury in a crash. It can literally be a lifesaver.

If you are lucky enough to have a recreational cycling or racing club nearby, you will find riders who are generous with advice about bike selection and riding. Just remember, if you start with a racing club, they'll ride harder and faster than you may be used to. Don't be discouraged if you can't keep up at first. Put in the miles and you'll improve. There's no way around it, cycling is a sport that takes a lot of training time. John Howard suggests: "If you really want to learn how to ride a bicycle, park your car permanently and commute."

Cycling Workouts

There's no substitute for long hours in the saddle to help build endurance and develop your cycling technique. You'll want to work on cadence, spinning at 80 to 90 rpm. You will also want to work on speed, spending at least one day a week on intervals. Carol Hogan's regular routine includes a ten-mile warm-up, followed by an intense ride for a specific time or distance. At first, her interval training consisted of riding as hard as she could for one minute, riding easy for three or four minutes, then riding hard again, and repeating this five times. As she grew stronger, she did longer fast rides with shorter rest periods in between.

Dennis Haserot, the 1982 National Veterans Time Trial Champion, suggests a training program for a triathlon bike race that includes doing intervals once or twice weekly to build speed and strength. His version of them consists of riding ten one-mile stretches or five five-mile stretches at maximum intensity.

How much you want to train on the bike depends on your goals. If you are already a fairly accomplished cyclist but want a new challenge, you may wish to try one or more of these three-month schedules prepared by Carol Hogan and Dennis Haserot. The first will prepare you comfortably to compete in a Tinman (one-fourth the distance of the Ironman). Completing the second schedule will prepare you for a half-Ironman. Completing all three schedules will prepare you for the Ironman.

First Three Months
Sunday: 30 to 35 miles, riding hard.

Monday: 20 miles, concentrating on spinning the pedals fluidly; an easier ride but include some hills.

Tuesday: 25-mile time trial, using the same course each time; keep a record of your time each week in your training log.

Wednesday: 20-mile ride with three minutes on/three minutes off intervals in middle of ride.

Thursday: one hour on indoor trainer to equal 20 miles. (This is optional. You may prefer to take a rest day.)

Friday: 20 miles with a local cycling group (if possible) in a paceline or same as Wednesday.

Saturday: 15 to 25 miles, riding easy.

Your total weekly mileage should be between 145 and 160 miles, enough to stress your body, build up your strength, and improve your cycling form.

Second Three Months
Sunday: 50 to 60 miles, riding hard.
Monday: 25 miles, spinning with hills.
Tuesday: 25-mile time trial; use the same course each time and keep log.
Wednesday: 30-mile ride with ten intervals, each two minutes on/two minutes off.
Thursday: 1½ hours on indoor trainer to equal 30 miles. (This workout is optional; take a rest day if you need one.)
Friday: 25 miles, group riding in paceline or same as Wednesday.
Saturday: 25 to 50 miles, long steady distance. Your total mileage should now average between 210 and 240 miles a week.

Third Three Months
Sunday: 75 to 100 miles, riding hard.
Monday: 35 miles, spinning with hills.
Tuesday: 50-mile time trial; use the same course each time and keep log.
Wednesday: 35-mile ride with one minute on/one minute off intervals.
Thursday: two hours on indoor trainer to equal 40 miles. (This is an optional workout; take a rest day if you need one.)
Friday: 45 to 60 miles or same as Wednesday.
Saturday: 20 plus miles, easy.
By now, you can ride 300 to 340 miles easily.

A Beginner's Running Schedule

When running, the whole musculoskeletal system in the lower body is going to take a pounding that a cyclist's legs are not accustomed to. This means stress on the connective tissue around the knees, for example. The best way to prevent injury is to begin with a run/walk program and workouts that last only about a half hour each. The first time out, run as long as you can comfortably—that is, without becoming too winded to carry on a conversation. Let's say you can do that for about 15 minutes. Divide that figure in half to determine the duration of the periods of continuous running in your next workout.

The next time you go out, run for 7½ minutes, then stop and walk for about 3 minutes. Repeat that sequence twice more to complete your half-hour workout. That way you will run enough to strengthen your heart but not enough to strain your muscles.

This pattern of stress-recovery is adapted week to week. As you grow stronger, increase your running time and slightly decrease your walking time. For example, the second week you may run for 8½ minutes before stopping to walk. This time, walk only for a couple of minutes before resuming running. Do this sequence three times for your half-hour workout. The following week you may extend your first two periods of running to 10 minutes each and end with a shorter run. With the next increase in length of your run, the number of sequences should be reduced to two. Eventually, you will be able to run for 30 or 40 continuous minutes, at least three times a week. At that point you are ready to start working on distance.

Advanced Training

When Carol reached the point where running 30 to 40 minutes was not a hardship, she began following a more intense running schedule. Beginning with a base of 16 miles, she increased her distance by about 10 percent every week, although the increase was a bit more rapid in the beginning. At least once a week, she also worked on her speed and strength in coaching sessions.

Carol's first week of intense running went something like this: Sunday, 7 miles; Monday, rest; Tuesday, 4 miles; Wednesday, coaching session; Thursday, rest; Friday, 5 miles; Saturday, rest. Week two went like this: Sunday, 8 miles; Monday, rest; Tuesday, 5 miles; Wednesday, coaching session; Thursday, rest; Friday, 6 miles; Saturday, rest. By increasing her mileage 10 percent a week, her schedule in the seventh month looked like this: Sunday, 20 miles; Monday, 6 miles; Tuesday, 10 miles; Wednesday, coaching session—intervals, sprints, etc.; Thursday, 7 miles; Friday, 11 miles; Saturday, 6-mile time trial.

Carol was fortunate in accomplishing this dramatic increase in mileage without injury. You can do this, too, providing you watch for the signs of overtraining.

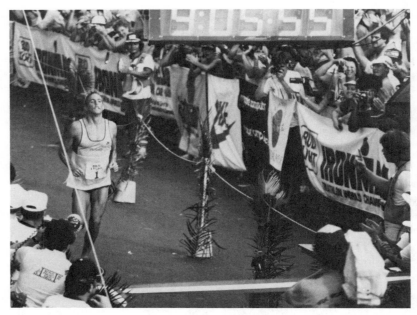

Photograph 4–7. Dave Scott crossing the finish line at the end of the marathon in the 1983 Ironman.

As Carol admits, following her training program will not guarantee you'll place in the top ten in a triathlon. You may even decide against competing, but winning a triathlon or even competing in one is not the most important benefit of multisport training. The main benefit is the feeling of strength and independence that such training will give you. You will find that to be more valuable than the fleeting glory of participating in even the most prestigious race.

Credits

The information in this book is drawn from these and other articles from *Bicycling* magazine.

"Introduction" Glenn Kranzley, "A Safe and Sane Way to Train," *Bicycling*, March 1982, p. 29.

"Shaping Up through Diet and Exercise" Susan Weaver and Bruce Hildenbrand, "Are You at Your Ideal Riding Weight

Now?" *Bicycling*, April 1981, pp. 54–55; Konrad Kail, "Spring Shape-Up," *Bicycling*, April 1984, pp. 35–38.

"Start Your Spring Training Indoors"   Tracy DeCrosta, "Getting a Jump on Your Spring Training, Indoors," *Bicycling*, January/February 1982, pp. 43–45.

"Don't Let Those Minor Aches Become Major"   Jeff Paulsen, "Injury Prevention—and What to Do When Minor Aches Become Major," *Bicycling*, June 1983, pp. 56–62.

"Put Your Legs in Good Hands with Self-Massage"   Ed Pavelka, "Self-Massage: Put Your Legs in Good Hands," *Bicycling*, July 1982, pp. 20–24.

"Weight Training as a Way to Prevent Injuries"   Tracy DeCrosta, "In Praise of Weight Training," *Bicycling*, January/February 1984, pp. 24–27.

"Training for the Beginning Racer"   George Liolios, "Training for the First-Year Racing Cyclist," *Bicycling*, May 1981, pp. 22–25; Fred Matheny, "Here's How You Can Get Into Racing," *Bicycling*, March 1982, pp. 30–33.

"Preparing to Ride Your First Century"   Walter K. Ezell, "Tackling the First 100" and "Training-at-a-Glance," *Bicycling*, September/October 1983, pp. 51–53 and 55–58.

"Embracing the Discipline of the Double"   Brooks McKinney, "Life in the Next Century" and "Training-at-a-Glance," *Bicycling*, April 1984, pp. 49–53 and 51–52.

"Total Fitness through Cross-Training"   Glenn Kranzley, "Totally Fit: The Benefits of Cross-Training," *Bicycling*, November/December 1983, pp. 28–32.

"Why and How to Cross-Train"   Carol Hogan, "A Multisport Training Manual," and Ray Hosler, "A Sporting Chance: A Comeback through Cross-Training," *Bicycling*, November/December 1983, pp. 32–45 and 42–44.

Photographs

Patrick Agnew: photo 2–2; Carl Doney: photos 4–2, 4–3, and 4–4; Peter French: photos 4–5, 4–6, and 4–7; T. L. Gettings: photos 1–2, 2–3, 3–1, and 3–2; Mitchell T. Mandel: photo 3–3; Alison Miksch: photo 2–7; Ken Redding: photo 2–1; Patty Seip: photo 3–4; Christie C. Tito: photo 1–3; Sally Shenk Ullman: photos 1–1, 1–4, 2–4, 2–5, 2–6, 2–8, 2–9, 3–5, 3–6, and 4–1.